I've Lost My WHAT???

I've Lost My WHAT???

✦

A Practical Guide To Life After Deafness

With a Foreword by Bill Graham Co-founder of the Association of Late-Deafened Adults

by
Shawn Lovley

iUniverse, Inc.
New York Lincoln Shanghai

I've Lost My WHAT???
A Practical Guide To Life After Deafness

iUniverse books may be ordered through booksellers or by contacting:

iUniverse
2021 Pine Lake Road, Suite 100
Lincoln, NE 68512
www.iuniverse.com
1-800-Authors (1-800-288-4677)

ISBN-13: 978-0-595-30661-9
ISBN-10: 0-595-30661-6

Printed in the United States of America

Dedicated to Bill Graham
and
the Association of
Late-Deafened Adults
for helping me see that
"life after deaf"
is no fantasy.

Contents

ACKNOWLEDGEMENTS

As anyone who's ever been masochistic enough to write a book can tell you, it's not a solo act, even when there's just one name after "by" on the front cover. <u>I've Lost My WHAT???</u> is no exception, so before you get to the good stuff in the book, I want to take a minute to thank everyone who helped make it a reality.

At the top of my thank you list is ALDA co-founder Bill Graham, who not only provided a warm and literate foreword for this book, but also offered intelligent feedback on many of the issues the work discusses. Bill is a truly impressive and inspirational person, and I'm proud to call him my friend. As they say Bill, "you the man."

I also want to thank Mary Clark, who has served as the head of the Association of Late-Deafened Adults (ALDA) twice, and was its president while I worked on this book. She offered all sorts of advice and suggestions while I was preparing it, and repeatedly served as my sounding board for it. While I'm in "ALDA mode," I want to send a big hug to Lori Heir, who co-edited the *2002 ALDA Reader* with me and helped me spread the word about this book. My gratitude also goes to everyone who contributed material to this book or suggested issues it should discuss. Thanks Ken Arcia, Nancy Kingsley, Steve Larew, Kathy Schleuter, Robin Titterington, Carolyn Piper, Glenn Cimino, Lynn Karavitis and her son Adoni, Lori Heir, Mark Dessert, Curtis Dickinson, Michele Bornert, and Cheryl Heppner, many of whom were ALDA officers in the past or serve on the ALDA Board of Directors at present.

Finally, my biggest hug is saved for my loving wife and best friend Marvelous Mary, who constantly reminds me that while my ears may not work anymore my heart "deaf" initely hears the words of love we share.

A GOOD BUDDY

A FOREWORD
by
Bill Graham
Co-founder of the Association of Late-Deafened Adults

I first heard from Shawn Lovley in the Spring of 1991. I was president of the Association of Late-Deafened Adults (ALDA) at the time and editor of the organization's newsletter, *ALDA News*. I lived in Chicago, the 1987 birthplace of ALDA and home to one of the group's most robust local chapters, a city at center stage of the growing network of people who became deaf as adults. Shawn was way out on the periphery of the stage. He lived in a city in the middle of Georgia, a state slow to discover the joys of ALDA. In fact, Shawn was one of only two people in Georgia on the ALDA mailing list. The other was Robin Titterington, a late-deafened woman who referred Shawn to ALDA, eventually headed up the Georgia Interpreters Service Network, and became ALDA president.

Our correspondence began with letters. Shawn had been recently deafened by brain surgery. He found his deafness difficult to live with and didn't know where to turn. He had been head of the theater department at Wesleyan College in Macon and now he found himself without a job. He had surrounded himself with highly articulate hearing friends, and now none of them could communicate easily with him. Ironically, Shawn's wife Mary was a sign language interpreter, but Shawn only knew a few signs himself and had a hard time relating to deaf people who used sign language.

I immediately took to Shawn. I liked his honesty, his sense of humor, his love for words, and his desire to help people. Even while he himself struggled with his new life, he mused about whether his experience might somehow benefit others. We exchanged several wonderful letters and then I called him by TTY. I goaded him and his wife Mary to attend the 1991 ALDA conference (ALDAcon) in Chicago. That was the year we initiated the ALDAcon "buddy system," in which first-timers to the 'con are paired with ALDAcon veterans. The buddy system was designed to ease the inevitable anxiety of a newly-deafened person wading into a sea of hundreds of other deafened adults. I was Shawn's buddy at the 1991 ALDAcon.

I got to know him and Mary well that week. I liked their style. One evening we got turned away at the door of The 95th, an elegant restaurant at the top of the John Hancock Building, because Mary was wearing jeans. Instead of being embarrassed, insulted, or disappointed (we were all pretty hungry), we laughed it off and ended up at Gino's East, a much more casual pizza place several blocks away. We had a great time there — jeans and all — and the evening became one of our fondest memories.

Shawn and I have been in close touch ever since. I've watched his incredible journey as a late-deafened adult with amazement and respect. Not long after the 1991 ALDAcon, he and Mary moved to the Washington, D.C. area, home to Gallaudet University and a large signing community. Shawn began to volunteer at Gallaudet's National Information Center on Deafness (NICD), gaining access to massive amounts of information about deafness and deaf people. He became the NICD's resident "expert" on acquired deafness, and won the university's "Volunteer Rookie of the Year" award for the 1992–93 academic year. He also began to write for *ALDA News* and eventually wrote for numerous other publications around the country. He also wrote two books before penning this one, and in 1993 won a playwriting competition at the New York Deaf Theatre with a humorous one-act play about late-deafness. His sign language skills improved dramatically too, and soon he was surrounded by highly articulate deaf individuals.

Shawn's journey continues to lead him to new areas of growth and discovery. His columns and articles have appeared in more than 30 periodicals, and he writes about late-deafness for a bi-monthly hearing-related newsletter and an on-line magazine. Once a self-professed "techno-dunce," he now regularly surfs the Internet, collecting items of interest and inspiration to share with his e-mail friends, many of whom he met through ALDA. He has played a major role in establishing electronic chat groups for late-deafened adults, and helped found ALDA-Potomac, serving as the editor of that chapter's monthly newsletter for several years. He was also elected to the 1996 national board of directors of ALDA, working closely with ALDA president and long-time friend Robin, and then served as ALDA treasurer in 2004.

Although he started far off in the wings, Shawn Lovley's courage and perseverance have brought him to center stage in the late-deafened world. In this book, Shawn shares much of the information and insight he has accumulated on his journey. The book serves as a valuable resource for all late-deafened adults, their families and friends, and professionals who work with late-deafened individuals. For people who are new to deafness, it will be an especially good buddy.

I'VE LOST MY WHAT???

✦

An Introduction

One Friday morning a while ago, the telephone rang at 7:15 — a bit early, no doubt, but not all that unusual. My wife Mary (or as I call her "Marvelous Mary") had to leave for work around 7:45 that day and she has at least two friends who sometimes try to catch her before she heads out the door. I imagined (correctly, it turned out) that the call was for her, so I let the phone ring until our answering machine picked up, because Ms. Marvelous was in the shower.

Why didn't I just pick up the phone and take a message? Well, I wanted to, but there's a little problem. See, I'm deaf. So I use a teletypewriter, better known as a TTY, which is a telephone device used by deaf and hard of hearing individuals. If someone calls me and doesn't use a TTY, he or she hears a lot of beeps from my TTY and nothing else. So when Mary's home, I don't answer the phone. I let her do it.

I'm not a typical deaf person either, although I doubt there is any such thing. I grew up hearing, and was 30 years old when I lost the use of my ears (except to keep my glasses in place) in December of 1990. I wish I could tell you that I've since become a sign language whiz or a speechreading expert, and that communication isn't a big problem for me anymore. The truth, though, is that my sign language is still thoroughly mediocre, my speechreading is even worse, and I now have a voice that can be really hard to understand because of the brain tumor that left me deaf.

My hearing loss isn't just a physical issue either. It's also had a powerful impact on my thoughts and feelings. It's hard (to put it mildly) not being able to hear voices or sounds after doing so for four decadess, and although I've found great joy in certain aspects of my post-hearing life (and never would have discovered many of them if I hadn't gone deaf), I can't escape the longing that I sometimes feel for my lost hearing and all it allowed me to do.

I also feel stuck between worlds, a sentiment that's quite common among late-deafened people. While I'm definitely not hearing anymore, I don't think like a

1

culturally Deaf person either. I'm sort of caught in the middle. I suspect that's true for most late-deafened people too. We're certainly not "hearies" anymore, but we're not like those who were born deaf or lost their hearing at a young age either. We're late-deafened. So it's for those people — which, according to statistics, make up a large portion of the American deaf population — that I've written I've Lost My WHAT??? The pages that follow provide the kind of information that late-deafened people are hungry for — assistive devices, the psychology of late-deafness, communication choices, television and telephone use after going deaf, the Americans with Disabilities Act, post-deafness relationships, legal aspects of deafness, cochlear implants, and hearing aids. It's the kind of book I wish had been around when I lost my hearing.

I'm not a scholar or an academic, and although I've done my share of research over the years, you won't find a lot of statistics or scientific facts about hearing loss in this book. Instead, it's meant to provide practical information about issues related to late-deafness. The book's goal is to make post-deafness life a lot easier for you or a loved one.

I'm also convinced that each late-deafened person has to find his or her own way of living after going deaf. Contrary to what some extremists claim, I don't believe there's any one approach that's "right" for all late-deafened people. So I've Lost My WHAT??? focuses on practical information on several topics rather than telling you the "best" way to live after losing your hearing.

Words, Words, Words

A few comments about the language used in this book are appropriate here.

"Late-deafened"

The Association of Late-Deafened Adults defines a late-deafened person as someone who loses some or all of his or her hearing post-lingually and requires visual cues to understand spoken words. That's a good definition, although I've Lost My WHAT??? takes things a little further. This book is intended to serve as a resource not only for those who were deafened after learning to speak, but also for those who grew up hearing and made major decisions regarding employment, social life, and personal relationships before their hearing loss occurred. It's also meant to provide information for people who were born deaf or lost their hearing at a young age and grew up using an oral rather than manual mode of communication in their everyday lives. The words "deafened" and "late-deafened" are used interchangeably in this book.

"Deaf" and "deaf"

You may have seen the word "deaf" spelled with both a "d" and a "D" in various publications. In case you're a little baffled by that, "deaf" refers to a physical condition — the inability to hear — while "Deaf" denotes a specific cultural identity. Those who were born deaf or lost their hearing early in life, attended a school for deaf persons, and rely on sign language as their primary means of communication, are often called "Deaf," while late-deafened people are usually referred to as "deaf." Several organizations, individuals, and publications use the "d" and "D" distinction to identify the respective groups, so don't be confused when you see both spellings in this book.

"Speechreading" versus "Lipreading"

The chapter about communication talks about deaf people who communicate orally and try to understand what others say without sign language. In the past, this process was known as "lip-reading," a term some late-deafened people still use. I find it rather inaccurate, however, because when deaf people try to understand someone's speech without help from sign language they do much more than read lips — they evaluate the speaker's facial expression and body language, as well as the environment in which the words are spoken. Reading lips is merely one part of the process of trying to understand what's said. So I use the word "speechreading," which seems to express more accurately what really happens. As a result you'll find that word, and not "lipreading," used in this book.

"Sign language" and "ASL"

Many late-deafened people who use sign language or are learning to do so refer to it as ASL, the abbreviated form of the name American Sign Language. The visual language most late-deafened people learn, however, generally isn't ASL. It's Pidgin Signed English (PSE), a name many people find offensive, Conceptually Accurate Signed English (CASE), or Signed Exact English (SEE), the latter two of which are often used by new signers. PSE, CASE, and SEE follow English grammatical rules and sentence structure, and are based on the spoken language most Americans use. ASL, by contrast, is a language in and of itself, with its own word structure and grammar. While the visual language most deafened people learn after losing their hearing use signs that are common to ASL, they usually learn some kind of English-based sign language, not ASL. As a result, the terms "American Sign Language" and "ASL" generally aren't used in this book, except to describe a specific language that most late-deafened people know little about. Instead, this book uses the term "sign language" to denote the type of gestural language deafened people generally use to communicate.

"Hearing-impaired"

Finally, the term "hearing-impaired," used a few years ago in an effort to be "politically correct," is no longer acceptable to many Deaf, deaf, and hard of hearing individuals or the organizations that serve them. There are certain people who still use the term, but it's extremely vague (is a "hearing-impaired" person deaf, Deaf, hard of hearing, or what?) and many individuals find it offensive. In her article "Don't Call Me Hearing-Impaired," late-deafened author Carolyn Piper wrote "being described as hearing-impaired is both grating and vaguely demeaning — a denial of a very real and important part of me." Some individuals use the term in private conversations to describe themselves, but you shouldn't use it to define anyone else without their permission, and you definitely won't see it in this book.

Now, Let's Get Started

Ready, set, go! I don't expect I've Lost My WHAT??? to answer all of the questions late-deafened people, their loved ones, or their workmates have about the world of acquired deafness. And while I consider myself more than a little fortunate to share my post-deaf life with a wonderful woman who happens to be an interpreter for the deaf (I married her before I lost my hearing — how's that for "foresight"?), my journey into deafness was one I had to take largely by myself. You probably will too. So don't be afraid to explore, experiment, succeed, and fail once in a while. That's just "life after deaf."

I'd also love to hear readers' thoughts on the subjects covered in this book. I'm planning companion books to I've Lost My WHAT??? about post-deaf romance, humor, and relationships with family and friends, and want to hear your thoughts on those subjects. You can send mail to me in care of the publisher, e-mail me at Shawn_Lovley@Yahoo.com.

ASSISTIVE DEVICES

Going deaf as an adult can be — to put it mildly — really scary and frustrating. Fortunately, there are all sorts of assistive devices we can use to help us function as fully as possible after a hearing loss, and make our post-deafness daily lives productive and satisfying.

The number of assistive devices that can help late-deafened people grows almost daily, so don't be too surprised if something you've read or heard about recently isn't listed in the following pages. If you want to stay current on what assistive devices are available, talk with a representative of one of the agencies mentioned in the chapter "A Resource Resource" to get the details on an assistive device you're interested in that isn't mentioned here. Although it naturally doesn't include all the devices available today, the following list will give you a good idea of what sort of items are available and how much you should plan to pay for them. The price estimates provided are accurate as of the summer of 2003, although they'll certainly change over time. So it's a good idea to visit a store that sells hearing-related items, look through some appropriate catalogues, or do an on-line search using a word like "hearing" to find out what's available and get current prices.

When you buy an assistive device, it's important to be able to return it, exchange it, or have it repaired easily. For many people, that means buying it locally. That's not always possible or desirable, so if you prefer or need to buy an item through a catalogue, over the telephone, on-line, or from a provider in another state, province, or country, be sure to get all the information you need about warranties, returns, and repairs before you fork over your dough.

It's also important to remember that assistive devices are exactly that — they're meant to help you live as well as possible with a particular disability rather than eliminate it. Use the ones that help you as much as possible after you go deaf, and remember that properly processing the information you receive is a lot more important than simply hearing it correctly.

So you won't have to fire up your computer or jump in your car right away, here's a list of some of the most popular assistive devices that are available today. New assistive devices appear all the time, so — as I said above — the following list isn't meant to be exhaustive. The items you can get your hands on will also differ from provider to provider, as will the prices for each of them.

Personal FM Systems

After losing some or most of their hearing, many individuals learn about FM systems, which amplify a speaker's voice for all listeners. By contrast, personal FM systems are meant to serve a single individual. They're light (usually two pounds or less) and easy to use. The speaker wears a transmitter, while the listener uses a small receiver and earphone to hear what's said. Personal FM devices, like all FM systems, amplify the speaker's words so they're easier to understand. They also minimize background noise so the listener can more easily understand what's being said. Most personal models use two standard — not re-chargeable — AA batteries. You should expect to pay about $650 for one.

Personal Amplifiers:

Closely related to personal FM systems are personal amplifiers. If you're late-deafened and have lots of residual hearing, but need amplification in order to understand voices, there are a number of personal amplifiers that can help. The following information comes from just one such amplifier, *The Pocketalker Pro*®, but will give you a good idea of the kind of assistance is available and the kindof options personal amplifiers offer. A small personal amplifier, *The Pocketalker Pro*® amplifies sounds in one-on-one communication and when listening to a device like a television. It also reduces background noise, making it easier to hear in noisy environments. It uses a pair of alkaline AA batteries, although you can also buy an adapter for it. *The Pocketalker Pro*® usually costs about $179, although a deafened friend told me she recently that she got hers on sale for $149.99.

TTYs

The chapter "That Phone Thingy" talks about telephone use by late-deafened people, and discusses TTY's (teletypewriters), which were later called TDD's (for "telecommunication devices for the deaf") or TT's (for "Text Telephone") and then TTY's again, in depth. Whatever you call them, though (most people say "TTY" now), a TTY is a device that you can use to talk by telephone with others who use a TTY or with hearing people through a Telephone Relay Service. If you're looking for a TTY, you have all sorts of choices. Basic non-printing TTY's usually cost between $225 and $400, while fancier models that offer printing and other options go for as little as $375 and as much as $800.

Combination TTY and Voice Telephones

Speaking of TTY's...Virtually all of the people I talk with on the phone have a TTY. Like many late-deafened people, though, I'm part of what my wife and I jokingly call a "mixed marriage:" I'm deaf, but she hears just fine, as do most of the people she talks with on the phone. So she usually uses the telephone in the traditional way. You might think separate phones or phone lines are the only answers for couples like us, but there are a number of combination telephones that meet the needs of both hearing and deaf people. They usually cost between $175 and $250.

Compact TTY's

If you're looking for a TTY you can take with you when you travel, there are numerous portable models available that can be used with a telephone or connected to a telephone line. Their keyboards (and hence, their keys) are usually much smaller than those on a traditional TTY, but travel models are generally markedly lighter than those meant for home use. Prices usually run from $200 to $375.

Voice Carryover Telephones

Many late-deafened people still have good voices after their hearing calls it quits, and like to use them when they're making telephone calls. If you're one of them, you might want to consider getting a voice-carryover (VCO) phone. You place VCO calls through a Telephone Relay Service (TRS), which is talked about in detail in the chapter *That Phone Thingy*, and you speak for yourself while a TRS communication assistant types what the other party says so you can read it on your TTY. VCO phones generally go for about $185.

Amplified Telephones

If you can still use the telephone without a TTY after your hearing loss, but want one that provides amplification, there are several different models available.

Many of them allow you to designate how loud or soft you want the voice on the other end of the line to be. Cordless amplified phones are also available. Many offer a handset that's hearing aid-compatible, a neckloop, or a patchcord jack for a cochlear implant. Expect to pay between $80 and $200 for one.

Voice/TTY Answering Machines

Closely related to the question of telephones in a household with both hearing and deaf residents is the issue of telephone answering machines. Hearing people can understand regular voice messages just fine, but late-deafened people's phone messages have to be in text form if they're going to be of any use to them. The solution? Get an answering machine that accepts both text and voice messages. There are a number of different kinds available. You should expect to pay about $325 for one.

Caller ID Machines

One of the greatest frustrations for many telephone users is not knowing who's calling when the phone rings. That can be particularly frustrating for deafened people, who often can't use the phone in the usual way and often end up with no text when they answer a call with a TTY. The answer? A caller I.D. machine. It displays the number and name a call is coming from, the time and date it was received, and allows users to modify entries as needed. There are also several models that can identify whether a call was placed by voice telephone or TTY. Caller I.D. machines generally cost between $17.50 and $20.00

Pagers

In addition to the various kinds of telephones available to late-deafened people now, there are also several different types of pagers, which are small devices that can be used to deliver text-only messages to other pagers (and in some cases, an e-mail address). Pagers that also deliver graphical images are being developed as of this writing. Pagers, which easily attach to one's clothing or belt, are usually quite light in weight (half a pound or a pound is common), have become very popular among late-deafened people, and you'll see lots of them in use wherever late-deafened folks gather. Pagers can be set to vibrate, blink, or make a sound when they receive a page, although deaf people usually choose the vibration option. Prices for paging service and options in pager hardware vary considerably.

Some providers offer free pagers if you subscribe to their service for the sending and receiving of pages (usually between $15 and $35 a month depending on how many pages you send and receive). If you plan to buy a pager (the free ones often aren't of a very high quality) you should expect to pay somewhere between $150 and $200.

Hearing Dogs

They might seem a little too cuddly to be considered assistive devices, but hearing dogs can be exactly that. When they hear a sound such as a ringing telephone, a knock on the door, and lots more, hearing dogs visually indicate it. The cost of training hearing dogs varies considerably, and it's sometimes paid for (partially or in full) by donors. Check with your state or province to see what's available. You can also look in *A Resource Resource* for general contact information.

Decoders

Decoders, which are devices that you can attach to a television in order to read closed captions, are becoming hard to find, because for several years now U.S. law has required new televisions with a screen that has a diagonal measure of 13 inches or more that are sold in the U.S. to have a built-in decoder. If you have a decoder in your TV but haven't used it yet, just play with your TV's menu and you'll probably be able to adjust your set to activate yours. If you have an older or smaller TV, you can usually buy an external decoder from a provider of hearing-related products for $90–$125.

Baby-Cry Alarms

There are a number of sound-based alarms on the market that provide some kind of noise when a baby is crying. Those aren't of much use to deaf people, however. Fortunately, there are several alarms that respond to a baby's cry with a flashing light, which makes them perfect for late-deafened parents. A number of individuals with hearing problems also use baby-cry alarms to provide a visual alert when something like an aural smoke detector goes off. Prices for visual baby-cry alarms vary from provider to provider, but usually run about $40.00.

Visual Smoke Alarms

If you're looking for an actual smoke alarm to alert you when there's a fire, however, you should know that most homes and apartments built today come with smoke alarms that provide both visual and aural signals when activated. If you buy or live in an older house, however, and it isn't equipped with smoke alarms that provide visual alerts, you can buy one and install it yourself. Expect to pay between $55.00 and $170.00 for one, depending on your house's wiring.

Doorbell and Knock Lights

There are also alarms that will blink or light up when someone rings your doorbell or knocks on your door. Rather than relying on your ears to tell you when you have a visitor, you can let your eyes do it. That's especially useful for late-deafened people when they're expecting a delivery — particularly one that needs to be signed for — or having a repair person come to fix something. You should expect to pay somewhere between $30.00 and $95.00 for one.

Vibrating Alarm Clocks

If you need an alarm clock to rouse you from la-la land but can't use a regular one because of a hearing loss, you can get one that vibrates at the time you desig-nate. Just enter the time you want to wake up, put the clock in your pillow case, and your pillow will shake at the time you've chosen. There are also alarm clocks that allow you to wake up to a loud buzzer — which can be helpful if you have sufficient residual hearing — or cause a lamp you attach to them to flash at the time you designate. There are also specialty alarm clocks that feature a large col-ored or lighted display for better visibility. Vibrating alarm clocks generally cost between $50 and $75.

Watch Alarms

Speaking of time and vibrating alarms…A late-deafened woman recently told me how much she loves her watch, because it can be set to vibrate at any time she chooses. Regular watches are generally no problem for late-deafened people who want to know the time because the information they provide is visual rather than aural. Watches with vibrating alarms, however, are especially helpful for deaf individuals who are on a tight schedule and need a reminder when it's time to head out. Prices for watches with vibrating alarms vary, although you should plan to pay somewhere around $80 for a basic model and $200 to $400 for a high-quality one.

Communication Linkage Devices

If your deafness is accompanied by a voice that's difficult to understand, you might want to get a communication linkage device that lets people know what you're saying. You simply type what you want to say on its keyboard and the device "talks" for you with the male or female voice you choose. At least one model also offers an optional telephone kit that allows you to make Voice Carry-Over calls through a relay service (relay services are discussed in the chapter *That Phone Thingy*). The units usually cost about $1400.

Modems

You may be familiar with the term "Modem," which is an acronym for "Modulator Demodulator." A modem is a device that converts data from digital computer signals to analog ones, which are then sent over a cable or phone line. You'll need one to send and receive e-mail or to "surf the net" (computer-speak for browsing the Internet). Many computers built today come with internal modems, although if you need to buy an external model, expect to pay anywhere from $80 for a very basic personal one to $350 for a top-of-the-line business unit.

The Internet

Originally used as a network to facilitate contact between organizations and agencies involved in military activity, the Internet has become very attractive to both industries and individuals in recent years because it's a major source of information and facilitates interaction between people. Late-deafened individuals are particularly fond of the Internet because it allows them to gather information and interact with others via text — so they don't have to worry about their inability to hear. Figuring out how to use the Internet may be a challenge for you, especially if you're a "techno-dunce" like me, and you might want to ask a computer whiz to show you how to get started with the Internet (teenage nephews and nieces seem to be quite adept at technical things like making computer behave).

In order to use the Internet you'll need an Internet Service Provider (ISP). Talk to friends or family members to find one that's right for you. Most ISP's include e-mail service with their Internet access, which can cost anywhere from nothing (advertiser supported) to $25 or more per month. You can also opt for DSL (based on Asymmetric Digital Subscriber Line technology) and other forms of high-speed Internet service, which provide very fast e-mail service and Internet "surfing." The cost is approximately $55–65 a month, although that varies from area to area and because of the various options you choose. High Speed Internet service usually uses a cable of some sort rather than a telephone line, so you can use the phone and be on-line at the same time without having to get a second telephone line.

Fax Machines

Another good means of communication for late-deafened people, although its popularity has declined markedly with the growth of e-mail in the past few years, is the facsimile (fax) machine. Fax machines allow the information on various documents to be transferred from one location to another via a telephone line. Some newer computers contain programs that let you send and receive faxes with them, although you can also buy an external model for anywhere between $80 and $300.

Fax-Modems

Closely related to both fax machines and external modems are fax-modems, devices that connect to a computer and telephone line and allow users to send and receive faxes and e-mail or browse the Internet. Many computers come with internal modems that allow you to do those things, although if you need to buy an external model you should expect to pay somewhere between $50 and $100.

Sign Language on a Compact Disc

If you'd like to use your computer rather than a dictionary in book form to learn sign language, you can pick up a Compact Disc (CD) that will let you do that. Most sign language programs on a CD are very complete, and users can usually choose the speed at which the sign for a particular word or phrase is presented, which comes in very handy as your skill level and comfort with sign language increase and you want to see signs at a faster pace. CD's containing sign language dictionaries are usually accompanied by a hard-copy version of the dictionary, thus making studying sign language without a computer easy. They cost about $50.

On-line "Chat"

A popular means of interaction for late-deafened people is electronic "chat," which allows people to interact with one another on-line via a computer and modem. Various on-line "chat" programs are available, and most of them can be downloaded for free of charge from the Internet, then easily installed and used to "talk" with others online. Two of my favorites are AOL's Instant Messenger (usually called "AIM") and ICQ (for "I seek you").

DON'T MIND ME:
The Psychology of Late-Deafness

The previous chapter talked about some of the many changes late-deafness brings into people's lives, and provided information about various assistive devices we can use to help us handle the practical challenges of going deaf: instead of using the telephone like we used to, we get a flashing light to let us know when someone's calling, buy or borrow a TTY so we can "talk" to others on the phone with it; we miss many of the words on television after we lose some or all of our hearing, so we use a decoder and read captions; we install a visual system to tell us when someone rings the doorbell or knocks on the door, and a device that flashes when the smoke alarm goes off or the baby cries. And on and on.

Some of the greatest challenges we face when we go deaf, though, are in the psychological arena. Fortunately, there are numerous books, articles, and video-tapes out there that talk about the psychology of deafness, and tell the stories of people who live life to its fullest with little or no hearing.

There's a catch, though. Those stories are almost all about people who were born deaf or lost their hearing at an early age and didn't have to make a major adjustment to a new life without sound. Losing your hearing as an adult, how-ever, makes you do exactly that. So in this chapter I want to look at the psycho-logical aspect of an adult-onset inability to hear, and talk about various coping strategies that can help you — or a loved one — navigate the sea of post-lingual deafness.

I'm not a psychologist, and what I've learned about the thought processes of deafened people comes from my own A.D. (After Deafness) experiences and more than a little input from my late-deafened friends. Pay attention to what applies to you in the pages that follow, and feel free to ignore the rest or modify it to fit your own needs and interests. If you'd like to look at the psychology of late-deafened individuals in detail, I strongly recommend a book that does exactly that — Deafened People: Adjustment and Support. Written by two late-deafened adults, Kathryn Woodcock and Miguel Aguayo, this very impressive book focuses primarily on the mental aspect of hearing loss, and may contain information that can help you live as fully as possible after you go deaf.

I also want to point out something important about deafened people searching for greater mental health. Traditional psychotherapy and counseling can be a great help to many people, but most mainstream therapists will know very little about deafness, and even fewer will understand the particular challenges of being late-deafened. So while I certainly don't discourage late-deafened people from seeking out a therapist, individuals who've lost some or all of their hearing as adults shouldn't be surprised if the counselor they're considering or working with simply doesn't "get it" when it comes to hearing loss or the particular needs and concerns of late-deafened people. Deafened people make up a large portion of America's deaf population, but the understanding of their particular concerns is beyond the ability of most therapists, even those who work with individuals who have some kind of hearing difficulty.

It *Does* Get Easier

Remember that biblical phrase "This too shall pass"? That's definitely true of the pain and frustration people experience when they lose their hearing. I belong to an on-line list for late-deafened people called "LDA Chat" (see "A Resource Resource" to learn more about it) that focuses on issues of interest to late-deafened adults, and we regularly get postings from new members who are dealing with a recent hearing loss. They're almost always confused and depressed, and wondering how they'll cope with their newly-silent world. While I've been deaf for more than a decade, and have had plenty of time to adjust to a life without sound, I still remember how depressed and frightened I was when my hearing called it quits back in 1991. If you're new to deafness, I want to assure you that it does get easier to cope with being deaf as time goes on. In his foreword to this book, ALDA co-founder Bill Graham writes about how lost I felt after I went deaf. That's a serious understatement! I was terrified and thoroughly depressed, and I didn't know anything about living in a world without sound. With the help of ALDA and my wonderful wife, though, I learned how. It will be the same for you.

It was also just a matter of time. After a while, my inability to hear simply became a part of me. So if you're new to deafness, and feeling blue because you can't hear anymore, know that the anguish of hearing loss fades as time goes on. It won't be easy to deal with your hearing loss at first, and the sadness you feel after your hearing calls it quits will probably never disappear completely. Most of the emotional pain acquired deafness causes, though, *does* pass. As time goes on you'll develop new interests and find new friends, which will help you realize that living a life with acquired deafness <u>does</u> get easier as time goes on.

It's Not Just You

It's also important for late-deafened people to remember that they're not alone in their grief over their hearing loss. Their family members and friends are sad about it too. Mine sure were. Although they never said it outright, it was pretty easy for me to see that my family and friends were deeply distraught when I went deaf. Suddenly, someone they'd known for years was sort of a closed book to them. They couldn't share the little "chit-chat" of everyday life with me any-more, or talk easily with me about something weighty that was on their minds. That really hurt both them and me. It got worse too. As time went on my voice became increasingly difficult to understand. That's usually not a problem for late-deafened people, but it was one of the "gifts" of the brain tumor that left me deaf. As a result, others couldn't always understand me. Both my loved ones and I did a lot of bluffing (a subject I talk about in the chapter about communication), but there was simply no denying that both them and me were deeply saddened by the fact that the easy communication we'd known for years was gone.

It's also important to remember that others' reaction to a hearing loss by someone they care about varies from person to person. It will range from accep-tance to panic to denial and include everything in between. Some people will readily accept the "new you" while others will feel — and often tell you — that you should get a powerful hearing aid or cochlear implant. Although they don't usually say it outright, some people believe the ability to hear again will make you more like the "old you." While I can certainly understand their desire for that, it's much healthier to do what's right for *you* rather than them (a subject talked about in more detail in the chapters about family and friends and cochlear implants).

Don't Sweat the Small Stuff

Probably the most important step you can take after your hearing runs off is to ask yourself if something you have to deal with is really all that important. Yes, many things in life are significant, and your hearing is one of them. But there are also a lot of things that deafened people (like everyone) worry about that don't merit raised stress levels. When you feel frustrated because you can't hear some-thing, it's a good idea to ask yourself if it will really matter to you a week, a month, or a year down the road. If the answer is "no" (and most times it is) make a conscious choice to let go of any pain and frustration it might have created for you and get on with your life.

It's also a good idea to ignore your negative feelings whenever possible. A thought is, often, simply that — a personal perception. It's usually just a creation of your mind, not a fact. Rather than allowing it to make you unhappy, why not simply refuse to let it upset you? I'm not talking about denying the thought's existence. Acknowledge it, and then simply ask yourself if it's really worth your time and energy. If it's not — and many of the things we worry about aren't — don't fret about it. One of my favorite t-shirts offers a couple of "rules" that seem particularly important to remember when we feel blue — "Rule 1: Don't sweat the small stuff; Rule 2: It's all small stuff." That seems like good advice for all people, regardless of hearing ability. Deafness may not be "small stuff" to you — it sure isn't to me — but my t-shirt reminds me of a very wise observation William James made several years ago: "The greatest discovery of my generation is that a human being can alter his life by altering his attitude."

A Difference or a Deficit?

Not sweating the small stuff doesn't mean you ignore things, though. The problems acquired deafness causes are very real, and ignoring them won't make them go away. In recent years, the "difference not deficit" model of deafness — which says that the inability to hear isn't a "deficit" at all, but just makes people "different" — has become popular among certain individuals and groups, particularly Deaf people and the organizations that support them.

In some ways, this makes great sense, especially for those who are culturally Deaf. After all, who would miss something they never had or don't remember because they lost it when they were very young? It would hardly be a deficit. A Deaf woman, in fact, once told me "Deafness is great."

I don't think many late-deafened people feel that way about their hearing loss, though. For most of us, our hearing is a significant part of our lives, and the loss of it is traumatic. Late-deafened people who claim otherwise are probably trying to convince themselves of that as much as anyone else.

To argue that acquired deafness isn't really some kind of deficit reduces the importance of sound, and seems to say that hearing isn't all that important, or that the loss of it isn't significant enough to be considered a major problem. Sorry, but it <u>is</u> important, and while I don't plan to stop enjoying my life because

I've gone deaf, I want to face my deafness and the fact that I have to live my life without hearing now. Only then can I get on with living.

I also wonder what embracing the "difference not deficit" model of deafness means in financial terms. If we want to publicly proclaim our support for it and still accept the economic benefits given to people because they're deaf, aren't we being a bit hypocritical? For example: if we argue that deafness is really just a difference and not a deficit, doesn't that imply that deaf people should give up the financial benefits — such as reduced transportation fares — that the inability to hear sometimes brings? You'd think so, right? Yet many of the same people who consider deafness no more than a "difference" are the first to accept that sort of help. Can we really have it both ways?

Another question: if acquired deafness isn't to be considered a deficit, why do organizations like the Association of Late-Deafened Adults exist? One of the major goals of the group is advocacy for those who lost their hearing post-lingually, and while there are no doubt lots of organizations that people just can't get too excited about (would you get very worked up about a group that urged people to visualize whirled peas?), I don't think ALDA is one of them. The group fills a very real and important need, and we minimize the role of organizations like it if we embrace a "difference not deficit" philosophy with regard to acquired deafness.

In a way, it all comes down to the need to accept rather than ignore or deny our deafness. Although "acceptance" has different meanings for different people, I agree with its general concept. Until we late-deafened people accept the fact that we can no longer hear, the opportunity to keep growing and changing will be limited. Isn't part of accepting our deafness acknowledging that a major hearing loss — never any fun for anybody — is something more than just a "difference"?

Stress

My wife and her sister both have t-shirts that say "All stressed up and no one to choke." That's a great play on the old expression "All dressed up and nowhere to go." I usually laugh out loud when I see them. Late-deafened people, unfortunately, often feel "all stressed up." It's difficult to feel at peace when your ears no longer work, particularly after being able to hear for years. When you go deaf, you're deprived of all sorts of practical information, and the easy interaction with others that you've grown used to becomes a thing of the past.

One solution to stress that many late-deafened people opt for is to find a counselor or therapist to help them. You may find such an approach particularly helpful, although, as I said before, it may be difficult for late-deafened individuals to find a counselor they can communicate effectively with or who will understand their particular concerns.

Fortunately, there are a number of things you can do yourself to eliminate stress or keep it to a minimum. The root to all of them, of course, is to "chill out" and consciously decide not to let things stress you out. A while ago I read an intelligent and amusing book by Loretta Laroche entitled Relax, which talks about the need to lighten up rather than cave into stress. I won't deny that stressful events are an inevitable part of life, especially when you're late-deafened, but the book's subtitle — *You May Only Have a Few Minutes Left* — definitely got it right. When you're confronted with something potentially stressful, ask yourself if you'd get upset about it if you knew you only had a few minutes of life left. You'll probably find that in most cases whatever has stressed you out simply isn't worth being upset about.

An especially good way to avoid extra stress is to simply breathe. You may be wondering how breathing could possibly help. After all, we do it all the time, and it's no big deal. Well, this little activity can make all your tension go away. Just breathe deeply several times, or consider doing some yoga or meditation, both of which are centered around breathing. If you feel like you don't have the time for extended breathing or meditation, or just want a quick burst of refreshment, simply take a single long, deep, relaxing breath. You'll be amazed at how much better that will make you feel.

If you do have time for meditation, there are all sorts of instructional books and pamphlets on the subject, so you won't lack for information. Until you get your hands on one, here are some basic guidelines to follow:

- If possible, set aside a room or spot in your house dedicated solely to meditation. You can also find a place outdoors that makes you feel peaceful and relaxed, and use it for meditating.

- Wash your hands and face or take a shower before you meditate.

- Don't eat too much before you meditate, since that tends to make you feel sluggish and tired. You want to be energized and alert when you meditate.

- Whether sitting on a chair, the floor, or the ground, it's important to keep your back straight during meditation. Many people who meditate believe that the energy meditation produces flows up and down the spine, and stress the importance of meditating in a way that creates a straight pathway for it. Lying down is also a good way to keep your back straight, although it often makes you fall asleep.

- Breathe slowly, steadily, and deeply while you meditate. Create an atmosphere of peace and awareness in yourself. Some people chant or burn candles while they meditate, and others simply sit or lie down calmly and breathe. The choice is yours. "Watching" the breath while breathing in and out is traditional, and is particularly helpful for beginners.

- Try to remain focused on your breathing during meditation. Stop conscious thought as much as possible.

- At the end of your meditation session, simply open your eyes slowly and return to the real world. Some people bow in gratitude and give thanks to the universe at the end of a meditation session, although that's certainly not required.

- Learning to meditate takes time. Don't expect to master it overnight. You may find your thoughts wander when you meditate, which is totally normal for everyone who meditates, especially beginners. When that happens, simply focus on your breathing and the relaxation that meditation can provide.

My friend Carolyn was deafened more than 25 years ago, and used to be deeply upset about losing her hearing. Now, however, she sings a very different tune. She meditates all the time, and the sense of calm and warmth she brings to everything she does and to all her relationships is truly impressive.

Sorry For What?

Not long after I went deaf I learned that some Deaf and deaf people believe you should *never* say something like "I'm sorry, but I'm deaf." They feel that deafness isn't something to be apologized for, that saying "I'm sorry" for being deaf is extremely negative, and unnecessarily lowers your self-esteem. That makes a lot of sense to me. After all, I hardly chose to be deaf, and my inability to hear doesn't define me. I don't see my hearing loss as some kind of insurmountable obstacle that I should apologize for. But there's a catch. When I say "I'm sorry, but I'm deaf" or something similar, I'm not so much apologizing for the fact that I can't hear as much as expressing my regret that my deafness often makes communication between me and other people difficult. For instance, if I'm checking out at a store and the cashier says something to me while looking down or away from me, I'll often say something like "I'm sorry, but I'm deaf" and ask for a repeat. There are a few people who simply ignore my statement or say something like the dreaded "it wasn't important," but the vast majority of them are more than happy to repeat themselves or write out what they've said so I can be sure I've understood it. That allows me to hang onto something much more important than my hearing — my connection with other people.

Denial

I often joke that denial isn't a river in Egypt, and although I like to tell myself that's pretty amusing, the reality is that denial can be a significant problem for many late-deafened people, who often spend a lot of time and effort denying their hearing loss, especially when they first go deaf. They refuse to acknowledge that they can't hear anymore, that their lack of hearing has affected their lives significantly, or that they really need to do something more than simply paying closer attention to other individuals' speech.

Unfortunately, many late-deafened people also don't want terms like "handicapped" applied to them, and are afraid that if they admit their loss to themselves, it will make their disability real. In fact, one deafened man I know who lives in a state where his deafness entitles him to a placard that would allow him to park in disabled parking spaces refuses to accept one. Although he doesn't say so outright, he seems to believe that accepting the placard would mean he's handicapped, and he doesn't want to acknowledge that. It's better for his mental health to hunt around for a parking space and walk the extra distance required after he finds one than to admit he's disabled and entitled to special consideration because of that.

Initial denial of a hearing loss isn't always a bad thing. Rather than throwing up their hands in defeat, many newly-deafened people simply refuse to accept the limitations deafness places on them. Sometimes people who deny a hearing loss develop skills when they first go deaf, and continue using them after they accept their loss. For example, not long ago I read about a deafened man who continued to direct plays in mainstream theaters long after his acquired hearing loss made it difficult for him to understand his actors, and now he uses the skills he developed in those days of directing mainstream theater to direct plays at various theaters for the deaf.

Unfortunately, denial often leads to very real problems. It delays the process of accepting your hearing loss, and makes it more difficult to recognize who you really are now. It strikes me as much healthier to tell yourself after you lose your hearing that you're deaf now and then get on with living as fully as possible within the parameters your hearing loss creates.

Denial isn't restricted to people who lose some or all of their hearing either. Some parents, family members, and friends of late-deafened people use it too. Recently, a late-deafened woman told me that although she was extremely hard of hearing as a youngster, her mother didn't want her to wear hearing aids. Her mom often denigrated the "ugly" free hearing aids her daughter was entitled to, and regularly implied that being deaf was awful. As a result, the daughter grew up thinking deafness was terrible, and her adjustment to a world without hearing, when she became a citizen of it, was slow and painful. The mother, who is now in her 80's, has also developed a severe hearing impairment herself over the past few years. She claims that she hears just fine, though — people simply don't talk loud enough. Talk about a serious case of the "denial isn't a river in Egypt" syndrome!

From Denial to Acceptance

The good news about denial is that it's often a temporary state. The amount of time late-deafened people spend in denial varies considerably, although they usually go through several of the following stages, and finish at the best one of all — acceptance of their new world.

1. *Denial of a hearing loss.* This first step is quite common among late-deafened people. It's sometimes evidenced by their tendency to speechread without doing so consciously, or opting for training in speechreading rather than sign language. Many deafened people feel that because they've always communicated orally in the past they should continue to do so when their hearing leaves, and that learning to sign would be an admission of their hearing loss — a step they don't want to take.

2. *Anxiety.* Many late-deafened people read about Deaf children having trouble learning to read or mastering some other important aspect of life, and become convinced that the old expression "deaf and dumb" is about being stupid rather than mute. They fear that having gone deaf they'll somehow lose the knowledge they acquired when they were hearing, or lose the ability to keep learning.

3. *Depression.* Many late-deafened people ask themselves pointless rhetorical questions such as "why me?" after their hearing leaves, and spend lots of time on what's been jokingly referred to as the "pity pot." Their

inability to hear leaves them feeling upset and depressed, and they wonder if a life without hearing is really worthwhile.

4. *Anger.* Several late-deafened people I've spoken with or read about go through a stage where they think "This isn't fair. I don't deserve this!" They refuse to see that — as a beloved t-shirt of mine says — "shiitake (a kind of mushroom) happens," and that there's no logical explanation for it. So they get angry about the "shiitake," over which they have absolutely no control.

5. *Guilt.* Although this is more common among parents of deaf children than adults who lose their hearing, many late-deafened people also feel their deafness is the result of something they "did wrong," such as not taking the "right" antibiotics or not getting to a physician quickly enough. Relatives of deafened people feel this way at times too. A deafened man once told me that his mother regularly "beats herself up" over his hearing loss, as if she were somehow responsible for it.

6. But then — the best step of all — *Acceptance.* This stage can arrive quickly or slowly, and depends a lot on both your own attitude and the people you socialize with. In a way, I was fortunate, in that my wife is an interpreter for the deaf, so I was able to meet all sorts of deaf people through her after I'd lost my hearing, and none of them felt their deafness was anyone's "fault," or that it diminished their worth as people. Seeing that made my transition to a silent world much easier and faster.

I realize, however, that late-deafened people can take a long time to reach the stage of acceptance. A big help in speeding the process is learning everything you can about hearing and hearing loss, and maximizing your contact with other late-deafened people. Whether you talk with them about acquired deafness or some other aspect of life isn't important — what matters is that you feel a genuine connection with them and that you both see beyond each other's limitations.

Gallaudet University president I. King Jordan, who was deafened at the age of 21 by a motorcycle accident, often says "Deaf people can do anything but hear." In a way, he's right — deaf people can do all sorts of things even if they can't hear, and Jordan has helped them see that deafness doesn't have to be an obstacle to happiness or success. On the other hand, however, I look at Jordan's statement as sort of an exercise in denial. Yes, there are plenty of things people can do if they're deaf, but there are also a lot of things that the inability to hear prevents folks from doing. It strikes me as much more realistic (and mentally healthier) to accept the fact that deafness imposes certain limits on people and to move on from there.

A case in point: In his book <u>Tuesdays with Morrie</u> author Mitch Albom recounts his weekly visits with his former college professor, Morrie Schwartz, who was dying of Amyotrophic Lateral Sclerosis (better known as ALS or Lou Gehrig's Disease in honor of the famed baseball player who died from it). By the middle of Albom's account there are many things Schwartz can't do for himself anymore. In one of his ensuing "classes" with his former student, Schwartz says it's important to realize what you can and can't do. Wouldn't it make sense for late-deafened people to realize that too? When we see that our inability to hear means that there are certain things we can't do anymore we can move towards genuine acceptance of our deafness. Until we do that we're simply fighting reality.

Live in The Moment

Kids can teach us a lot about living in the moment — a skill most of us have as children but lose as we get older and start dealing with things like rent or mortgage payments, our children's tuition, or (when you're deaf) if you've properly understood what someone has said to you. A true story I read recently sums up the problem perfectly, and although the father and daughter in it are both hearing, it offers an important truth that applies to everyone, regardless of his or her hearing ability.

The father had hired a babysitter to watch his two-year-old daughter while he and his wife went out for the evening. The father and daughter were playing in her sandbox behind the house when the sitter arrived, and the youngster got very upset when she realized that daddy would be leaving soon. As the father stood up and prepared to go, the daughter let out an ear-piercing scream of disapproval. She wailed profusely and made it abundantly clear that she didn't want Daddy to leave. He did anyway. Shortly after Mom and Dad made their escape, though, the father realized he'd forgotten his car keys, and went back inside to get them. He peeked out his back door at the sandbox and saw his daughter smiling, laughing, and generally having a great time playing in the sandbox. It was as if the event with Dad was ancient history — or had never happened. The daughter was living fully in the present.

How often do we allow ourselves to do that? Yeah, the daughter may have been subconsciously manipulating her father (or consciously — kids can be pretty clever!) by crying and screaming when he prepared to leave. It seems more likely, though, that the youngster was simply voicing her strong objection to her father's departure, and when she realized it was inevitable she decided to enjoy the moment. Going deaf as an adult is sort of similar. You can moan and grieve about it, and you will certainly do that at first. In time, however, you need to accept the reality of your loss, and get back to living. Mark Dessert, who lost his hearing several years ago and is now the editor of *ALDA News*, put it perfectly:

> Life isn't fair or unfair; it's just life. When the rug gets pulled out from under you, get angry. Cry. Grieve. Take time to heal your wounds. But don't take too much time. Get back into life as soon as you can. We'll be dead far longer than we've been alive, so there's no time to waste.

<u>Courage</u>

Getting back into life after going deaf can require a lot of courage. After all, you've spent years as a "hearie," and you enter a whole new world when your ears stop doing their job. You can bet that's really scary, and the idea of facing your loss with courage can seem ridiculous, particularly if you don't consider yourself very brave.

You're probably braver than you think, though, and acting courageous might be just what you need. When you act brave, even when you don't really feel that way, it sort of takes you over, and you become courageous. It's tough to feel gutsy when you first start putting on a bold front, but in short order your actions will begin controlling your thoughts, and you'll think of yourself as a really brave person. Before you know it, real courage follows.

I speak from personal experience. A few years after a brain tumor took away my hearing, a friend told me I was the bravest, strongest person she'd ever met (I think she actually meant I was the "bravest, *strangest*" person she'd ever met — one little letter makes a big difference, huh?). I know for sure, though, that I wasn't too brave before my tumor showed up. In fact, I was really kind of a wimp. After my tumor was diagnosed, though, I decided to start telling myself that I was as courageous as could be, and in short order it became true. Now, more than a decade after the tumor was "supposed" to kill me (or so the statistics said) I've turned into a pretty gutsy guy. I'm not implying that I don't want to crawl into a hole and hide at times, because I sure do. Pretending I was courageous in the years after my diagnosis, though, helped make me that way. I bet it will work for you too!

It's also important to remember that being courageous doesn't mean you can't be scared at times. Once in a while your inability to hear will leave you frightened, but there's nothing wrong with that. It sure doesn't mean you're not courageous. As Mark Twain once said: "Courage is resistance of fear, mastery of fear — not absence of fear."

Getting Help

As gutsy as you may become after you go deaf, one of the most important things you can do to speed the recovery process is to look for help in adjusting to your new world. While I said earlier that it's difficult to find a psychotherapist or counselor that can provide meaningful help in your journey, the good news is that the principle element in that trip is help from someone you know quite well — yourself! It's no coincidence that ALDA offers a self-help workshop at its annual conference each year, or that one of the most popular organizations for hard of hearing individuals is called "Self-Help For Hard of Hearing People." Self-help is easily the most important step we can take after we lose some or all of our hearing, and usually one that precedes all others. I'm hardly a self-help "guru," but there are some simple, yet important, self-help steps late-deafened people can take to help make their transition to the world of deafness as painless as possible.

The first — and probably most important — step to take when you lose your hearing is to join a self-help group. My personal favorite is the Association of Late-Deafened Adults (ALDA), which has been a great help to me in navigating my post-deafness world. I encourage you to learn about the group if you haven't already done so. Check out the "Resource Resource" chapter to find out how.

Unlike other self-help groups that deal with hearing, ALDA focuses specifically on post-lingual deafness. Most of the group's leaders and the vast majority of its members are late-deafened, and lost their hearing after making choices about work, education, employment, romance, marriage, and parenting. There are also all sorts of ALDA members who are spouses or relatives of deafened people, as well as therapists, audiologists, doctors, and nurses who know, work with, or care for deafened individuals.

Whether you choose ALDA or some other self-help group, it's important to remember that "self-help" is exactly that. Self-help groups and their members can help you find your way, which can be especially hard to do when you first go deaf, but you should only count on them for a short period, and nothing more. While you can obviously enjoy interacting with the members of a self-help group for a long time, it's important to look to the organization itself to supply the tools and inspiration you need to allow you to do your own exploring and learning. Only you can really know what you need and want, and you should consult with an expert — yourself — on the subject.

You might ask why, if you're supposed to provide help for yourself, you should bother to join a group that focuses on self-help. There are lots of reasons. The most obvious one, of course, is that belonging to a group like ALDA will provide you with access to all sorts of important information about assistive devices and help you answer the practical questions that arise when you go deaf.

More important than that, joining an organization such as ALDA will allow you to work through the issues of going deaf with the help of people who've "been there and done that." Individuals who have personal experience with adult-onset deafness can provide information and help that's based on personal experience, which is usually much more helpful than the advice provided by a book or suggestions from an audiologist or counselor. People who've "walked the walk" of acquired deafness can provide the kind of honest feedback and emotional support that's often so hard for newly-deafened people to come by, and you should definitely avail yourself of it.

Closely related to that is the fact that virtually all members of ALDA are late-deafened, or are close to someone who's lost his or her hearing post-lingually. As a result, the group's members know what other ALDAns are feeling. That also means that everyone in the group, despite a severe hearing loss, feels normal with one another. Being deaf doesn't make them "different," which can be a big problem for late-deafened people who live and work in the mainstream world. For example, when you attend the annual ALDA conference your hearing loss isn't an obstacle to enjoying yourself or gathering important information. In fact, it's just the opposite. It makes you (to borrow the title of a popular *ALDA News* column) "One of us."!

If I had to sum up the benefits of a self-help group like ALDA, I'd put together a list like this:

- Members gain knowledge and information about a subject that's of great importance to them.

- The information ALDA provides usually comes from people who've "walked the walk" of acquired deafness rather than simply "talked the talk" about it. They've lived the experience of acquired deafness instead of just reading about it somewhere or knowing someone who's lost his or her hearing. As a result, members learn what's worked for others who've gone deaf, and realize it might help them too.

- Members gain motivation and confidence, and receive support, because they're surrounded by others who are dealing with the same challenge they are. Even better — they see them winning. That makes newly-deafened people feel they can win too.

- Being part of a self-help group allows members to evaluate their own progress via feedback from other members, and by sharing their experiences and feelings with individuals who've often been through the same thing they're facing.

- Members grow because they're able to help others. I've long believed that one of the greatest tools for personal growth is helping others. Belonging to a group like ALDA allows people to do exactly that.

Whether you join a self-help group right away, or some time down the road, there are all sorts of things you can do on your own to feel better about yourself, your relationships, and the world you live in. Here are just a few suggestions, none of which require the ability to hear. I hope you'll also come up with others that fit your particular situation, needs, and interests.

Develop a New Attitude

Both late-deafened and Deaf people can't hear, but they have very different attitudes about deafness. Although very few Deaf persons express sadness at being deaf (after all, they've been without hearing for most or all of their lives), late-deafened people often feel downcast about losing their hearing. If that describes you, it might help to develop a new attitude, which you can do if you follow these four steps of mourning for late-deafened persons, which were provided by a deafened individual with a Ph.D. in counseling:

1. Accept the reality of the loss. The loss isn't only real, but as far as we know, it will be with us as long as we live. In the words of Jordan: "Deafness is permanent. Deal with it."

2. Work through the pain of the loss. Being upset or confused about your hearing loss is absolutely normal. Let yourself go through the grief and pain that comes from going deaf. Then get on with your life. To quote one late-deafened woman: "At first, I was shattered. As I became more comfortable with my deafness and learned more, though, I accepted it, made my peace with it, and tried to learn from it."

3. <u>Adjust to your new work and play environments.</u> It will be an ongoing process, but you *will* get used to your hearing loss. In the words of one late-deafened man who went to college after going deaf, and graduated with highest honors, deafness is "just another part of my identity now."

4. <u>Emotionally re-invest your life in relation to the loss.</u> Do something positive after you lose your hearing. Whether this means working or volunteering for an organization you care about, going back to school, or doing something else important to you, remember that you *are* somebody. Do whatever makes you feel good about yourself.

Assertiveness

Lots of people confuse the word "assertive" with "aggressive" and think they mean the same thing. They don't! Aggressiveness is usually hostile and often violent. By contrast, assertiveness is simply understanding what you need or want and then doing whatever's necessary to make it happen, whether by asking for something or doing it yourself.

Late-deafened people are particularly prone to having problems with assertiveness. They don't want to risk offending others, and are afraid that if they're assertive they might do just that. As a result, they often spend lots of time suffering in silence because they're reluctant to accept their hearing loss and do things to lessen its impact on them. If they do accept it, they often don't want to risk annoying someone by asking for a simple accommodation. Other times they don't know what to ask for in the first place.

Fortunately, becoming assertive isn't difficult, as the following piece proves. In the 2002 edition of *The ALDA Reader* Nancy Kingsley wrote about her trip to the land of assertiveness after going deaf. I was so impressed with the piece that I asked Nancy if I could include it in this book, and she graciously said "yes." So here it is.

◆   ◆   ◆

Becoming Assertive About Communication Needs — A Work In Progress

by
Nancy Kingsley

For many years, I spent a lot of time suffering in silence because I was reluctant to acknowledge my hearing loss, didn't want to annoy anyone by asking for an accommodation, and/or didn't know what to ask for in the first place. As a result of this self-defeating approach, I sat through numerous events without knowing what was going on, feeling miserable and sorry for myself. This was the period when I compared my life to a beautiful dress with a large stain.

One day, as I was sitting through yet another lecture that I couldn't hear, I had an epiphany. It struck me for the first time that I, too, had rights — that there was no good reason why I should have to endure this kind of psychological torture solely for the purpose of blending in unobtrusively with everyone else. I whispered to my husband, "I can't hear — let's leave!" We were in the front row as usual, in order to maximize my ability to speechread, so we could hardly disappear unobserved. Mindful of this, my husband responded, "What about the speaker's feelings?" For the first time, I shot back, "What about <u>my</u> feelings?" So we got up and left, and from that moment on I no longer allowed myself to be trapped in a communicative black hole. It was a remarkably freeing experience.

During my voyage toward assertiveness, I encountered many obstacles and gradually learned to overcome them. At one disability-oriented event, the microphone was positioned directly in front of the speaker's lips, making speechreading impossible. After the speaker finished, I asked the conference coordinator to lower it so I could speechread the remaining speakers, whereupon she responded haughtily, "We have an interpreter!" I was so taken aback that it didn't even occur to me that I should have told her that not every deaf person understands sign language.

Fast forward to a more recent event, shortly after I received my cochlear implant and was able to use assistive listening devices. By this time, I was becoming better at speaking up for myself, but I hadn't fully arrived yet. At this particular event I had given the speaker my portable FM transmitter and was able to understand her well. Unfortunately, the pastor was sitting in the back of the room, interjecting comments at various points during her presentation. At first she brought the transmitter over to him when he spoke and he returned it to her when he finished. After awhile, however, she apparently tired of this, and from that point on I could no longer understand his comments. After she finished speaking and was returning my transmitter, I commented, "Do you remember when you stopped passing the transmitter to the pastor? Well, I was still deaf!" She got the message.

Although this was an improvement over my previous passivity, it was too late to correct the immediate problem. I had been inhibited from acting at the appropriate moment due to the taboo against interrupting an ongoing presentation, but this barrier also had to fall. The first time I spoke up on such an occasion was at a meeting of parents of deaf children, which made me feel relatively safe. The speaker had moved the microphone to a location in front of a window, causing his face to be in a shadow, and I called out for him to close the drapes so I could see to speechread. He immediately did so, and I felt the same flush of empowerment that had washed over me the first time I left a lecture that I couldn't understand. (Afterwards, an audiologist came over to tell me that I had role-played what she always tried to encourage her clients to do.)

Things got easier after that, and I even found myself able to be assertive about my communication needs at a program that wasn't related to disability or hearing loss. When one of the speakers (who knew that I needed him to wear my portable transmitter in order for me to hear him) ignored my effort to hand my transmitter to him when he came by to distribute papers, I thought he would come back for it before starting his talk. Unfortunately, he began addressing the audience while I was still sitting with the transmitter in my lap. So I rose, walked silently up to him, and handed him the transmitter. He understood and put it on, and I returned to my seat.

I've also learned that it's sometimes necessary to speak up more than once. At a recent small-group meeting, I gave my transmitter to the speaker, explaining that it needed to be passed along to anyone who had questions or comments. When she didn't follow through, I reminded her, and she said she would repeat the comments instead. To my surprise, though, she mouthed the words instead of saying them aloud, so I had to ask her to use her voice (she later told me she hadn't realized that she had turned it off). Everything went smoothly from that point on.

Requesting appropriate communication access was another important milestone (Thanks to the Americans with Disabilities Act, public accommodations and state and local governments are required to provide effective communication.). When my son received a Masters in Social Work from New York University, I arranged for the university to provide CART for me for the graduation, and being able to understand what the speakers were saying was a refreshing change of pace from my experiences at similar events in the past.

Finally, learning about various communication coping strategies was a big help. I've been able to improve my communication environment considerably by using these methods, such as asking for a door to be closed to eliminate background noise and taking the seat next to the window at a restaurant table so my companions' faces won't be in the shadows. I've found that politely explaining my needs has generally been sufficient (except for requests that require people to change their habits, a difficult challenge for most folks). The crucial factor is knowing what to ask for. My increased ability to be assertive developed in parallel with my increased self-esteem, which in turn was enhanced by my interactions with other late-deafened and hard of hearing people. As I've become more open about my needs, I've found it easier to get them met. If my life once seemed to resemble a badly stained dress, it now looks like I've found some pretty good spot removers!

◆   ◆   ◆

Depression versus Mourning

While Nancy's story is heartwarming and encouraging, the unavoidable fact is that many late-deafened people mourn their loss or become depressed when they can't hear anymore. Is there a "right way" to respond? What's the difference between mourning and depression?

The key to answering that question can be found in the difference in the definitions of the two words. One dictionary defines "mourning" as "the actions or feelings of one who mourns." "Mourn," in turn, is defined as "to feel or express sorrow, lament, grieve." "Depression" is defined as "low spirits, gloominess, dejection, sadness."

These definitions may seem pretty similar, but they actually reflect very different mindsets. Mourning is a natural result of any significant loss, whether it's your hearing or something else. When you mourn, you're simply grieving for what's gone. Eventually, you move past it. If you lost your hearing and didn't mourn about what had happened, the important people in your life would probably wonder just what your problem was.

Depression, by contrast, implies a deeper level of mourning. Recovery from it can be difficult, if not impossible. The mourning person expresses his or her sorrow for what has happened, faces it, and eventually goes on with life, but the depressed individual feels sadness at what's happened, and often doesn't ever get past that.

It's perfectly normal to feel grief over what's gone, and individuals who mourn sometimes become depressed. People can't make a conscious choice between the two, and when a late-deafened person becomes depressed, it may be necessary to seek some kind of professional help. If that describes you, get it. If, by contrast, you simply feel sad about your loss, allow yourself to feel that way for a while, remind yourself that's perfectly normal, and remember there's a whole world waiting for you after you go deaf. It doesn't know or care that you can't hear anymore. So get back into life. As the wonderful film *The Shawshank Redemption* says, "Get busy living or get busy dying."

Conclusion

Is there a bottom line when it comes to the psychology of late-deafness? I don't think so. I do know, though, that even if one exists I'm not the one to tell you what it is. As I said at the beginning of this chapter, I'm hardly an expert on the subject of psychology for late-deafened people. I do believe, though, that it's OK to rant and rave about your loss until you've achieved a full acceptance of it. The time will probably come when you'll accept your loss, but when you first go deaf you also need a chance to moan about what's happened to you. So share your feelings with those close to you, and if screaming, crying, or stamping your feet makes you feel better at first, then by all means do it. In many cases, the healing process can't begin until you allow yourself to grieve. Doing so can be an important first step towards inner peace. After you've done that you can move on and live fully in your new world.

Whatever you do, though, it's important to remember not to be ashamed of your hearing loss. To quote Jordan again: "It's part of me. Accept me. Accept my deafness."

Say What?: Communication for Late-Deafened People

One of the biggest challenges for late-deafened people is that of communicating after going deaf. When our ears no longer work like they used to we have to develop other ways to listen to the voices in our world, and that can lead to some real problems. There are a number of different choices we can make to help us do that, though, and in this chapter I want to talk about them.

As with many things in life, there's no right or wrong choice when it comes to communication. Choose what's appropriate for you, and don't be concerned about pleasing others or doing what they say you should do. I once read that you should never "should" on yourself, and that seems particularly true with regard to communication choices. Realize too, that while a specific form of communication may be appropriate for one situation, a different type might be more appropriate for another. The Association of Late-Deafened Adults has adopted a "whatever works" philosophy regarding communication, and I hope you'll do the same. Use whatever works for you whenever it's called for, and don't be concerned about choosing the "right" means of communication. The only "right" choice is the one that fits the particular situation, and suits your interests, needs, and abilities.

Sign Language

You may have seen people communicating with each other using sign language and wondered what it was or how it worked. To put it simply, sign language is a very expressive form of manual communication that uses hand positions, body language, and facial expressions to convey facts, thoughts, feelings, and ideas. Many deaf individuals use sign language as a primary tool for communication, and it's certainly not necessary to master it fully or sign quickly in order to feel at home with it.

As I pointed out in the introduction, there's a marked difference between American Sign Language (ASL) and the sign language most late-deafened signers learn. ASL is a language in and of itself, with its own grammar and word structure, and is usually only used in the Deaf community. Very few late-deafened people who sign use ASL. Instead, they usually rely on a form of communication that uses the signs of ASL but is based on the English they grew up with.

If that's not ASL, then what's it called? Well, there are several different forms of sign language used by deafened individuals. The most popular, though, is Pidgin Signed English (PSE), a name some people — as I also pointed out in the introduction — find offensive, and which uses signs from ASL in English word order. You may also hear about Conceptually Accurate Signed English (usually called "CASE") or Signed Exact English (generally referred to as "SEE") which, as the names suggest, are precise and detailed visual forms of English. SEE includes articles like "the," "a," and such, none of which are used in PSE or ASL. Sometimes it's difficult to find anyone who uses CASE or SEE, although a late-deafened woman (who's a *much* better signer than me) once told me that she's talked with several deafened people, particularly at the annual conference of the Association of Late-Deafened Adults, who use one or the other.

Late-deafened people who learn sign language do so at various speeds, and may fingerspell (spell manually) a word until they know the sign for it (if one exists). As deafened signers become increasingly comfortable with manual communication, and more aware of its vocabulary, the need for fingerspelling decreases. Fingerspelling is often especially challenging for deafened people to master, and practicing it both on their own and with accomplished signers can be extremely helpful.

The learning of various types of sign language has increased markedly in recent years, but it's important to remember that there are still many situations where late-deafened people have little choice in terms of what kind of sign language they can learn. For example, I recently met a late-deafened man who had to study ASL because the only way he could learn sign language was by working with a man who was born deaf, and whose principal means of communication was ASL. I've also learned, however, that most Deaf people are very patient with late-deafened people's (often flailing) efforts to use sign language, and don't have any hidden desire to spread the use of ASL. They simply want to talk with others who sign, whether they're Deaf, deaf, hard of hearing, or hearing, and whether they use ASL, PSE, or some other form of sign language.

Some late-deafened people develop enough skill in sign language to use interpreters for the deaf, who listen to a third party's spoken words and then translate them into sign language so the deaf person can understand what's being said. I'm a *little* biased in favor of interpreters (often called "terps") because my wife is one, but I also realize that many late-deafened people simply never learn to read sign language well enough to benefit from interpreters, who often sign quickly in order to keep up with the speech of the speaker they're interpreting. Rather than using an interpreter, many late-deafened people rely on various print-based forms of communication, which I discuss below. While they're usually markedly slower than sign language, they eliminate the risks of uncertainty and confusion that sign language can create.

Speechreading

In some ways, it's perfectly natural for late-deafened people to learn speechreading. The basic concept of speechreading — sometimes called "lipreading" — is straightforward: by watching the speaker's mouth and body, and considering the location and situation of the interaction, a speechreader can often tell what's being said. Many late-deafened people don't care for speechreading because it's quite unreliable, but if you can speechread well, it may help you retain your connection with the hearing world after you go deaf. While my own speechreading skills are quite limited, several late-deafened people I know speak very highly of it, and agree that the following elements are essential to the effective use of it.

- Choose a well-lit and quiet area whenever possible. Be sure to position yourself in such a way that you can see the other person's face well. Light from windows and lamps should illuminate the speaker's face, but not so brightly that it impairs the ability to see his or her lips, face, and body. If you'd like to improve visibility, you can change your position or ask the other party to do so.

- Whenever possible, know the subject of the conversation before it begins. You may want to ask the other person to write down a word or two about the topic before the discussion begins. This will be of great help, both in terms of understanding the subject and saving yourself some energy in figuring out what the other person is talking about.

- Many people who lose their hearing are left with a certain amount of residual hearing. If you're one of them, it can markedly improve your speechreading skill. In order to benefit from residual hearing as fully as possible, get yourself and the speaker to a quiet setting whenever possible.

- Speechreading well takes a lot of energy. Don't be afraid to limit the amount of time you spend doing it in a single session, and be sure to take breaks as needed. If you're tired, consider having the conversation at another time if possible. Fatigue — as many accomplished speechreaders will tell you — is a serious obstacle to speechreading effectively.

- Whenever possible, make sure you've understood spoken words correctly, particularly if the discussion includes specific facts you need to know, such as addresses, names, the time and place of a meeting, or details about a medicine you're supposed to take. Repeat significant things that have been said to you, and ask for important points to be written down for you.

- News is often the basis for many conversations, so it's important to keep up with current events as much as possible.

There are also several things a speechreader can ask a speaker to do in order to improve communication:

- Speak naturally. Many people who don't understand speechreading think they should slow down or shout in order to be more easily understood. The truth is just the opposite: speakers who talk very slowly or yell are actually considerably harder for a speechreader to understand than those who talk normally.

- Don't cover your face or mouth or turn your head away when you speak. Speechreaders need to see your face in order to understand you.

- Don't speak from another room or talk when the lights are out.

- Use facial expressions whenever possible, and try to make them match and reinforce what you're saying.

Sounds pretty easy, right? Unfortunately, speechreading can be difficult to learn, and doesn't work for everyone. There are several reasons for that —

- Speech and hearing professionals have estimated that about 60 percent of the sounds in English speech are either hard to see or invisible. For example, people can usually see p, b, m, th, and f on the lips but k, g, and ng are virtually impossible to speechread. In addition, many letters look similar. For example, it's difficult to tell "p," "b," and "m" apart when you speechread because they all look alike.

- In order to speechread effectively, you must be able to see what's said. That means the speaker has to face you, stand or sit a reasonable distance from you, and be in light that's bright enough (but not too bright!). Unfortunately, that often doesn't happen, unless you pretty much abandon spontaneity and give the other party very specific instructions.

- A person's ability to speechread is closely related to his or her knowledge of language and the various elements used in it — words, phrases, idioms, and speech patterns. People who know more than one language will probably find that they speechread best in the language they're most comfortable with. Those who speechread also find that reading speech that's spoken with a dialect or accent is very hard to decipher. This can make speechreading a real challenge for deafened individuals who move somewhere new.

It's important to remember that the ability to speechread is a skill some people are born with and some aren't. Certain individuals claim that anyone can speechread, but the truth is that if you weren't born with an inherent talent for it, you may never really be able to master speechreading, no matter how much you practice. So don't blame yourself if you don't speechread well. Your inability to do so may just be a matter of genes.

Cued Speech

Although it can be difficult to find other individuals who use it, Cued Speech is popular among some late-deafened people. What's Cued Speech? A sound-based visual communication system which, in English, uses eight handshapes in four different locations (called "cues") in combination with mouth movements to facilitate understanding. It's generally used to develop language skills in deaf or hard of hearing children, although some late-deafened individuals have benefitted significantly from it too.

How does cued speech assist communication? Here are a few of its most notable features:

- Through Cued Speech a late-deafened adult can have access to spoken English again — which means he or she can enjoy peer communication and — via a hearing person who "cues."

- If you want to learn a foreign language after losing some or all of your hearing, use of a Cued Speech interpreter will allow access to the language's precise spoken form.

- Cued speech is of special interest to late-deafened people whose primary language isn't English. It's based on the phonemes of any spoken language, and not limited to any particular one.

If you'd like to learn more about cued speech, I encourage you to contact the National Cued Speech Association (NCSA), a non-profit membership organization that was founded in 1982 for the purpose of promoting and supporting the use of Cued Speech. It raises awareness of Cued Speech and its applications, provides educational services, assists local affiliate chapters, establishes standards for Cued Speech, and certifies Cued Speech instructors and transliterators. You can contact the NCSA by writing to it at 23970 Hermitage Road, Cleveland, OH 44122-4008, calling (800) 459-3529 (T/V), e-mailing cuedspdisc@aol.com, or visiting its web page at http://www.cuedspeech.org/Cued_Speech_Discovery.html.

Print-based Communication

Not long after I went deaf I attended a sign-language camp in upstate New York. The other attendees were also new to deafness and/or sign language, so their signing and speechreading skills, like mine, were quite limited.

One evening after a day of classes, several of the students were sitting around talking. I forget the exact topic being discussed, but I do remember that there was no paper and pen or keyboard in sight. Although there was a lot of smiling and nodding going on, it didn't take me long to figure out that there was also very little comprehension happening. Some camp attendees were so determined to remain as "normal" as possible that they pretended to understand one another and overlooked a valuable communication tool which is especially useful for deafened people who don't sign or speechread — print-based communication.

The easiest and most reliable means to receive information when you first go deaf is through written text. How that happens isn't important. What matters is that you understand others and that they can follow what you're saying. That lessens the impact of your deafness on you and allows others to continue communicating with you.

Print-based communication can happen in several different ways. One of the most popular is with a pad and pen/pencil. You can also use a small erasable slate, where messages can be written with a special kind of pen and then easily erased with a sponge or eraser. Another great tool for print-based communication is the TTY. I don't mean for telephone calls either. Two people can sit next to one another with a TTY, type messages, and they'll appear on the screen of the TTY so they can be read. As she points out in the later chapter about romance for late-deafened people, my hearing wife and I do that all the time when one of us has something important to say and don't want to risk being misunderstood.

The same is true of computers. Use of them has grown tremendously in the past few years, and recently-deafened people can take advantage of everything computers have to offer, including e-mail and on-line chat. Perhaps even more important, computers can facilitate in-person communication. Simply type what you want to say into a computer, and it appears on its monitor so the other party can read it. Reverse roles, and — presto! — genuine interaction has taken place. Laptop computers are especially useful for communication that occurs outdoors or when you're indoors but away from a desktop model. Whether you use a lap-top or desktop computer, you can change the size, color, and appearance of the letters that appear on the screen, thus making them easier to read.

The computer-based approach to communication isn't limited to one-on-one conversations either. It can be used in group or meeting situaions as well. In many such settings Computer-Assisted Notetaking (CAN) is employed. CAN doesn't provide word-for-word transcription of every word said, but offers summaries of what's talked about, which are usually displayed on a screen that several people can see.

For situations where exact transliteration is required or desired, there's Communication Assistance Realtime Translation (CART), formerly known as Computer Assisted Realtime Transcription. Used in an increasing number of venues, including the annual conferences of the Association of Late-Deafened Adults and the National Association of the Deaf, CART is an adaptation of court reporting. The words of the speaker are typed into a computer by a highly skilled individual and appear on a screen so they can be read by everyone in attendance. CART can be expensive because of the pricey equipment and expert operators it requires, so it's often more costly than using professional sign-language interpreters. Nevertheless, it's a valuable resource for late-deafened people, who often aren't skilled signers or speechreaders, and prefer to use text-based communication to assure proper understanding.

Another option for late-deafened people looking for print-based communication is C-Print, which is a form of voice-to-text translation. It uses a typist with a computer that has a special program. C-Print's not as fast or complete as CART, but many colleges have started to use it for non-signing deaf students in the classroom. It requires special training and a specific computer program. If you'd like to learn more about C-Print, you can call 585-475-2809 (tty/voice), send an e-mail to CPrint@rit.edu, or head to the web site http://www.netac.rit.edu/.

Deaf Man's Bluff

The camp experience I described above unfortunately isn't all that unusual. Lots of late-deafened people don't want to accept their hearing loss or tell anyone else, especially strangers, about it. So they bluff, a process in which a deaf person pretends to be hearing or to have understood what someone else has said. Bluffing is something many late-deafened people do quite regularly. That's not too surprising. After all, individuals who've lost their hearing post-lingually have usually spent years as hearing people, and were able to understand what people said by paying only minimal attention to them. Going deaf, though, makes that virtually impossible. We want to continue to be "normal" after we go deaf, though — or at least appear that way — and asking for a lot of repeats, saying "what" frequently, or thrusting a pen and piece of paper at people so they can write out what they've said isn't the way "normal" folks communicate. So we bluff.

While bluffing can provide late-deafened people a modicum of short-term relief and comfort, it often results in long-term unhappiness and uncertainty. In some cases, it leads to outright disaster. Just imagine what would happen if a late-deafened person bluffed with his or her doctor or pharmacist and ended up following an incorrect course of treatment or was unaware of how best to take a certain prescription medicine. Talk about the potential for disaster!

Bluffing isn't restricted to deaf people either. As I said earlier, I have a pretty terrible voice now, and many hearing people have had to ask me to repeat or write down something I've said so they can be sure they've understood me correctly. Unfortunately, in lots of situations, hearing people clearly didn't understand what I've said, and instead of simply asking me to repeat what I'd said or write it down, they've bluffed that they understood me and then done something that was exactly the opposite of what I'd said. Fortunately, none of this bluffing has had serious consequences (so far, anyway), although it does provide a powerful reminder that bluffing is sort of a universal phenomenon.

Conclusion

As you can see, there are lots of communication alternatives available to late-deafened people, and you'll have many options after you lose your hearing. Don't be concerned about making the "right" choice, though. Just pick the one that's right for you, realize that different modes may be appropriate for some situations and not others, and — most important of all — don't be too concerned if you aren't an "expert" at one or more of them.

The Americans
With Disabilities Act

The Americans with Disabilities Act (ADA) is one of the greatest boons to disabled people that ever came down the pike. Several people have called it the "Emancipation Proclamation for Disabled People" because it protects all Americans who have a disability from discrimination in many aspects of life, including employment, housing, communication, and public services.

National awareness of the ADA is presently at an all-time high. A poll taken in 2002 found that 77 percent of Americans say they are aware of the law, a marked increase from the 67 percent recorded three years earlier. The news gets even better too: a massive 93 percent of those who know the law exists approve of it. The complete text of the ADA can be found in most libraries, and if you prefer to learn about the law from an electronic source, you can read the complete ADA and lots of other useful information at:
http://www.usdoj.gov/crt/ada/cguide.htm# anchor62335.

Although the ADA was landmark legislation that was well-publicized, particularly among the disabled, it can also be a bit confusing. So in the next few pages, I'll discuss the four titles of the ADA and their meaning for deafened people, as well as answer some questions regarding the specific reach and intentions of the act. While this information is accurate as of the time of publication, people interested in the law and what it means are encouraged to contact their lawyer, local deaf association, or city, state, or national government to get detailed information about the act.

Despite the law's general popularity, certain individuals and groups are currently working hard to limit the effect of the ADA on various businesses and institutions. Sometimes they succeed too. For instance, the Supreme Court recently ruled that recipients of federal funds, such as states and cities, can't be sued for punitive damages for violating laws that are tied to federal grants unless Congress expressly says so when it enacts laws that effect them. Other efforts to limit the ADA are also in the works, which seems to happen whenever U.S. politics move to the right. Since there's lots of confusion about what the ADA can and can't do at any time, it's wise to consult an individual or organization with special knowledge of the act whenever you have a question that's not answered here.

Before we can look at the ADA's meaning for late-deafened people, I want to put an important concern to rest. Some people are worried that deafness, because it's not visible, may not be covered by the ADA. If you're concerned about that, you can relax. The ADA considers deafness a disability, and serves to protect deaf people from many kinds of discrimination. So if you're anxious about losing your job or your home when your hearing goes south, rest assured that the law is on your side.

What the ADA Says

The Americans with Disabilities Act is divided into four sections, called "titles," each of which provides protection for disabled people in a specific area. Below is a description of what each title addresses and how the law can protect you at present.

Title I took effect on July 26, 1992 in companies with 25 or more employees. Two years later, those with at least 15 employees were also covered by it. Title I says that private employers may not discriminate against any disabled applicant or employee on the basis of that disability with regard to any condition or privilege of employment. Employers are required to provide a "reasonable accommodation" to any employee who "can perform the essential functions" of a job, provided it does not impose an "undue hardship" — meaning an unrealistic expense or difficulty — on the employer. For a late-deafened person, a "reasonable accommodation" may mean a TTY, reassignment to another position where hearing isn't essential, modified work schedules, restructuring of a job to eliminate its non-essential aspects, or an alteration of job-related examinations or training materials. Employers are also not permitted to choose qualified non-disabled applicants over equally qualified disabled ones on the basis of the latter's disability.

Title II of the ADA is particularly relevant to deafened people who have disabilities in addition to their hearing loss. It says that no disabled person can, by virtue of that disability, be excluded from, discriminated against, or denied the benefits of any department, agency, special purpose district, or any other instrumentality of a state or local government. To put it in plain English, a state or local government can't discriminate against anyone with a disability in its programs or services — whether or not those programs and services receive federal financial assistance.

Title II also focuses on accessible public transportation (air travel is excluded). Any new buses on a fixed route must be accessible, unless a public transportation authority can demonstrate that lifts are not available from qualified manufacturers. A public transit authority must also offer comparable special transportation services to those who cannot use standard transit unless provision of such services imposes an undue financial burden on the provider.

<u>Title III</u> of the ADA prohibits discrimination against a disabled person in the enjoyment of goods, services, facilities, and privileges in any place of public accommodation operated by a private entity or business — hotels, restaurants, doctors' offices, private schools, health spas, senior citizen centers, and so on. Private clubs and religious organizations aren't covered by Title III, and some doctors have attempted to avoid serving disabled individuals by simply refusing to accept them as new patients.

Title III also specifies that existing facilities be made accessible to disabled users, provided the required changes are "readily achievable" and don't cause undue expense or difficulty. Auxiliary aids such as TTYs, television decoders, visible emergency alarms, and so on must be supplied upon request unless this would impose an undue burden on the provider. Hearing dogs also must be allowed on the premises of all public accommodations, and new construction intended for use as a place of business must be made accessible to people with a disability.

<u>Title IV</u> is of special interest to late-deafened people who enjoy using the telephone. It requires the creation of a telephone relay service (TRS) in all states around the country. Discussed in depth in the chapter "That Phone Thingy," a TRS facilitates telephone contact between users regardless of their hearing ability by acting as the "ears" of a deaf or hard of hearing person talking by telephone with a private individual or business representative who's not using a TTY.

If you're not sure of exactly how the act applies to you or the company you work for, you might want to get in touch with one of the Disability and Technical Assistance Centers listed below. They're funded by grants from the National Institute on Disability and Rehabilitation Research, and are eager to help people who can benefit from them.

T=TTY, V=Voice, F=Fax

Region 1 —
Connecticut, Maine, Massachusetts,
New Hampshire, Rhode Island,
and Vermont

University of Southern Maine
Muskie Institute of Public Affairs
96 Falmouth Street
Portland, ME 04103
(207) 780-4430 (V)

Region III —
Delaware, District of Columbia,
Virginia, and West Virginia

Endependence Center of
Northern Virginia
2111 Wilson Blvd.
Arlington, VA 22201
(703) 525-3268 (V)

Region V —
Illinois, Indiana, Michigan, Minnesota,
Ohio, Wisconsin

University of Illinois at Chicago
University Affiliated Programs in
Developmental Disabilities
1640 West Roosevelt Road
Chicago, IL 60608
(312) 413-1647 (V/T)
(800) 949-4232 (V)

Region VII —
Iowa, Kansas, Nebraska, Missouri

Region II —
New Jersey, New York,
and Puerto Rico

United Cerebral Palsy Association
of New Jersey
345 S. Broad Street
Trenton, NJ 08908
(609) 392-4004 (V)

Region IV —
Alabama, Florida, Georgia, Maryland,
Pennsylvania, Maryland
Kentucky, Mississippi, North Carolina
South Carolina, and Tennessee

United Cerebral Palsy Association
S.E. Disability & Technical Assistance Ctr.
1776 Peachtree Road
Atlanta, GA 30309
(404) 888-0022 (V)
(404) 888-9006 (T)

Region VI —
Arkansas, Louisiana,
New Mexico, Oklahoma, Texas

Independent Living Research
Utilization/The Institute for
Rehabilitation and Research
2323 S. Shepard Blvd., Ste. 1000
Houston, TX 77019
(713) 520-0232 (V)
(713) 520-5136 (T)

Region VIII —
Colorado, Montana, North Dakota,
South Dakota, Utah, Wyoming

University of Missouri at Columbia
ADA Projects
4816 Santana Circle
Columbia, MO 65201
(314) 882-3600 (V)

Region IX —
Arizona, California, Hawaii, Nevada,
Pacific Basin

Berkeley Planning Associates
440 Grand Avenue, Suite 500
Oakland, CA 94610
(510) 465-7884 (V)

Meeting the Challenge, Inc.
3630 Sinton Road, Suite 103
Colorado Springs, CO 80907
(719) 444-0252 (V)

Region X —
Alaska, Idaho, Oregon,
Washington

Washington State Governor's
Committee
212 Maple Park KG-11
Olympia, WA 98504
(206) 438-3167 (T)
(206) 438-3168 (V)

Limits to the ADA's Reach and Efforts to Weaken It

Earlier in this chapter I mentioned that certain organizations and individuals have attempted to narrow the scope of the ADA. In case you need proof of that, you might want to know that a recent verdict forbids victims of discrimination from recovering punitive damages from organizations that don't have to abide by the ADA.

This verdict is opposed by many people because it may discourage legitimate discrimination cases in the future. There appears to be some truth in that assumption, because while the ADA says a lot about the illegality of discrimination, it doesn't provide a specific enforcement mechanism to prevent or discourage it. For instance, while it's illegal for a state or local government to discriminate against people with disabilities, they won't be punished for doing so unless someone takes them to court. That often takes lots of money, and many disabled people simply can't afford such an action, so the case isn't pursued. As a result, violators are free to continue discriminating without fearing punishment.

Another concern is that the Americans with Disabilities Act, as it currently stands, really supports lawyers who work on ADA cases rather than those who are protected by the law. For example, the settlement of a 1999 class action suit resulted in the University of California at Davis and the University of California at Berkeley agreeing to improve accommodations for people with hearing loss. The universities also agreed to pay each of five plaintiffs $10,000 each. Not exactly chump change, huh? Except.... The universities were also told to pay the lawyers' fees of $1,100,000 in the case. So the lawyers received more than 20 times as much money as the five plaintiffs combined. You can just imagine how a layperson without a disability (a huge majority of Americans) would feel about the outrageous costs of such cases, and wouldn't be too interested to know that students with less-than-perfect hearing now have better access at these two schools because of the ADA.

If you do decide to pursue your rights under the ADA, you should know that many lawyers often accept cases with the understanding that they'll get a percentage of any award as payment. That's very common in the legal world. Unfortunately, there's a little trick when it comes to the ADA. You can often only get compensatory damages from the kind of suits associated with the act, and they're generally considerably lower than punitive damages. So winning a case like that would mean less money for a lawyer. As a result, attorneys may be hesitant to accept a case if it only guarantees a percentage of a relatively small award that a plaintiff *might* win. So while the law forbids discrimination, it often requires the victim to pay for its enforcement. As a result, many individuals are discouraged from pursuing cases against organizations that violate the law.

Lawyers have another reason to hesitate when it comes to taking an ADA-related case — the chances of winning one. The Supreme Court recently reversed a lower court ruling that awarded $1.2 million in punitive damages to a paraplegic. The decision was unanimous, but only six justices joined in Justice Antonin Scalia's majority opinion. A concurring opinion warned that Scalia's written opinion was "sure to have unfortunate consequences." It agreed with the verdict, but wanted the case decided on narrower grounds.

The case wasn't immediately related to deafness. It involved Jeffrey Gorman, who was arrested in 1992 outside "Guitars and Cadillacs," a nightclub in Kansas City, Missouri, after he'd tangled with a club bouncer. Officers had strapped Gorman to a bench inside the police van for the ride to the police station, but on the way he fell, injuring his shoulders and back.

Gorman, who was convicted of trespassing, sued Kansas City police officials, claiming they had violated the ADA by failing to provide adequate means to transport a person with his disabilities. Gorman was awarded over $1 million in compensatory damages and $1.2 million in punitive ones, but upon appeal a federal district judge threw out the latter award. The 8th U.S. Circuit Court of Appeals later reinstated the punitive damages, and Kansas City police officials then appealed the case to the Supreme Court. An opinion is being awaited as of this writing.

The immediate relevance of this particular case to late-deafness may seem somewhat unclear. What it says about the ADA and its ability to protect disabled people, however, is frighteningly obvious.

Questions and Answers

In the years since its passage, the ADA has been the subject of much misunderstanding and plain old erroneous information. What follows are some common questions asked about the ADA and their answers. If you want to know more, or are interested in a particular subject, you can contact one of the regional ADA offices mentioned above or the government agencies listed in "A Resource Resource."

Q: *Who, specifically, does the ADA protect?*

A: All qualified individuals with disabilities and persons with a known relationship with a disabled person. The ADA defines an individual with a disability as anyone who has an impairment that limits him or her in some way with regard to significant life activities such as hearing, seeing, walking, breathing, learning, caring for oneself, and working. This definition includes persons with a history of cancer that's currently in remission, and those who have been diagnosed with mental illness. The ADA also prohibits discrimination against those who are regarded as having a substantially limiting disability even if they function "normally." For example, a seriously disfigured individual who is qualified for a job may not be refused that position on the basis of possible negative reactions by other employees or customers.

◆　　　◆　　　◆

Q: *Can an individual sue a business when he or she believes a violation of the ADA will happen, or does that person need to wait until the actual discrimination occurs?*

A: The public accommodations section of the ADA allows individuals to allege discrimination based on a reasonable belief that it is about to occur. For example, a person who uses a wheelchair may challenge the construction of a proposed shopping mall if it would not be accessible to wheelchair users. The resolution of such challenges before construction begins would allow modification of design plans to include these changes, which is far less expensive than making alterations after building has been completed.

◆   ◆   ◆

Q: *Does the ADA apply to the federal government?*

A: Not completely. The executive branch is covered by Title V of the Rehabilitation Act of 1973, which makes it illegal to discriminate in employment or services on the basis of disability. The ADA, however, does apply to Congress and other sections of the legislative branch.

◆   ◆   ◆

Q: *How does the ADA affect state and local governments?*

A: Title II of the ADA mandates that all facilities and services of these governments be accessible. Individuals can file complaints with federal agencies designated by the Attorney General or through private lawyers.

◆   ◆   ◆

Q: *Does the ADA cover private homes and apartments?*

A. In general, no. When places of public accommodation, such as doctors' offices or day-care centers, are located in private residences, however, the portions of the private residence that are used for that service are subject to the regulations of the act.

◆   ◆   ◆

Q: *The ADA doesn't cover air travel. Does anything?*

A: Yes. Air travel is covered by The Air Carrier Access Act [49 U.S.C. 1347 (c)].

◆   ◆   ◆

Q: *Some businesses claim the ADA is too expensive for them. But will they qualify for tax benefits to help them pay for compliance?*

A: Yes. The Internal Revenue Code was amended in 1990, and allows a deduction of up to $15,000 a year for any expense related to the removal of certain transportation or architectural barriers.

◆   ◆   ◆

Q: *How about late-deafened people shopping? Will a bookstore, for example, have to provide a sign language interpreter to communicate with customers who don't hear well?*

A: In most cases, no. Employees can generally communicate with customers who are deaf or hard of hearing with pad and pen.

◆   ◆   ◆

Q. *The ADA contains employment non-discrimination requirements. What specific practices are covered by it?*

A: Employers may not discriminate against disabled people in any employment practices, including hiring, firing, promotion, compensation, training, privileges, recruitment, tenure, leave, layoffs, and fringe benefits.

THAT PHONE THINGY:
Telephone Use After Going Deaf

When the device that allowed deaf people to use the telephone first appeared in the mid-1960s it was called a TTY, an abbreviation for "Teletypewriter." A few years later, a new name was developed — TDD, an acronym that stood for "Telecommunications Device for the Deaf." Then it became a TT, shorthand for the government-approved term "Text Telephone." A few years later, a late-deafened friend even jokingly dubbed it a TPT for "That Phone Thingy." While you probably won't run across the term "TPT" anytime soon, and both "TDD" and "TT" are still used in some places, in most quarters "TTY" is back in vogue.

Confused? Well, all these names (even "TPT") mean essentially the same thing — a machine often used with a telephone that employs text rather than sound so that deaf and hard of hearing people can talk by phone with friends.

History of the TTY

As many people know, the telephone was invented by Alexander Graham Bell over a hundred years ago. It allowed people to talk with one another, whether they were across the street or the country from each other. Today it's difficult to find an American home without a telephone in it, and it's essential for survival in business.

There was an ironic catch with this invention, though. For years the telephone, created by a teacher of the deaf who was a strong advocate for them, was inaccessible to many people with less-than-perfect hearing. Fortunately, this began to change when the TTY was invented. With the recent creation of telephone relay services (described later in this chapter), telephone access for deaf and hard of hearing people has taken another important step forward. Bell would be a very happy man indeed.

Research on the modern TTY, a type of telegraph machine that printed the messages it received in text, began in 1963, when deaf physicist Robert Weitbrecht and deaf orthodontist James Marsters started exploring ways in which deaf people could communicate by telephone. By 1964, Weitbrecht had developed an acoustic coupler that converted electrical impulses from a teletypewriter into sounds that could be transmitted over telephone lines. After these sounds traveled across telephone wires, the teletypewriter at the receiving end converted them back into electrical signals. They were then turned into text that showed up on the screen of the receiving teletypewriter. Now, just a few decades later, TTYs play a central role in the lives of many deaf and hard of hearing people. There's still plenty of confusion about them, so below is a brief explanation of what's in a TTY, what they do, and how they work.

What's In a TTY?

The Keyboard: All TTYs have a keyboard of some kind, which follows the lay-out of a standard typewriter or computer keyboard. Three-row keyboards gener-ally have the numbers 0–9 as uppercase characters above the letters QWERTYUIOP, while four-row keyboards usually offer more characters than their three-row counterparts, such as!, @, #, $, %, ^, _, and +.

The Display: TTYs provide some means of displaying in readable text the sounds they receive. Most have a single light-emitting diode that shows the text, which usually travels across the screen from left to right.

The Coupler/Modem: The TTY's coupler/modem converts outgoing electrical impulses into sounds that travel across phone lines, and changes incoming sounds into electrical impulses so they can appear on the TTY's display as letters. Some TTYs have rubber cups on them where a telephone receiver must be placed, while others have a "direct connect" feature, which means people can use them without a telephone. In addition, new combination TTY/telephone devices can be used for both TTY and voice calls, an important consideration in homes where deaf and hearing people use the same phone.

How Much Does One Cost?

Options and Prices: Many TTYs have optional features, such as memory, printing capability, a rechargeable battery pack, portability, and so on. You can also install special software that allows you to use your personal computer as a TTY. Your individual needs and interests will determine what special features you require. Prices range from about $150.00 for reconditioned models to $600.00 or more for sophisticated new TTYs. Ask the salespersons at the stores you visit in your hunt for a TTY plenty of questions before you buy one, and be certain the TTY you purchase suits your personal needs and preferences. If you're concerned about being able to afford one, many states offer programs that pay part or all of the cost of a TTY. Your state's deafness commission will be able to tell you more.

Using Your TTY

Placing a TTY call: After turning on your machine, place your telephone's receiver in your TTY's cups (if your TTY has a "direct connect" feature, that isn't necessary). Then dial or enter the number you wish to reach. A TTY usually has a light which tells you the status of the call you're making. A slow steady blinking after dialing indicates the telephone you've called is ringing. A flickering light means that the phone is being attached to a TTY. A rapidly blinking light means the number you've called is busy. When the call is answered, identify yourself and use the following TTY etiquette. Abbreviate or standardize common words. Many people also shorten frequently-used terms and don't use punctuation marks. Here are some common TTY abbreviations:

ASAP: As soon as possible	NBR or NU: Numbers
ASST: Assistant	OIC: Oh, I see
BIZ: Business	OFC: Office
BYE: Good-bye	OPR: Operator
CA: Communication Assistant	PLS: Please
CD or CLD: Could	PPL: People
CUL: See you later	PRO: Professional
CUZ: Because	Q: Question (sometimes used instead of a question mark)
DR or DOC: Doctor	R: Are
EDUC: Education	SD or SHD: Should
FIGS: Figures	SK: Stop Keying (ending a call)
GA: Go ahead	SKSK: Hanging up
GA SK: Ready to hang up	THRU: Through
HD or HLD: Hold	TMR or TMW: Tomorrow
ILY: I love you	THKS or THX: Thanks

IMPT: Important	U: You
LTRS: Letters	UR: Your
MISC: Miscellaneous	URS: Yours
MSG or MSGE: Message	XXXX: Erases an error
MTG: Meeting	

Interference: TTY calls are sometimes affected by interference, which can cause symbols, numbers, or nonsense words to appear on the screen. Tapping the space bar of your TTY sometimes eliminates this annoying jumble. In addition, when TTY users call people who have TTYs but don't normally use them, the sound this tapping makes tells them they're receiving a TTY call. Deaf people can also call a hearing person through a telephone relay service and let him or her that you'll be contacting him or her by TTY soon. Then there will be time for the hearing party to set up his or her machine.

Whose turn? : GA means "go ahead." It should be used each time you're done typing what you want to say, so the other person knows it's his or her turn to type.

Finishing a call: The person who wishes to conclude the conversation should type his or her final statement, a good-bye, and then the letters GA SK. The other person can then continue the call or simply type his or her good-bye followed by SK SK.

An example*:* A TTY conversation might go like this —

> Bob: Hello. Bob here. GA
> Lisa: Hi Bob. This is Lisa. How are you Q GA
> Bob: Hi Lisa. I'm fine thanks. How are you Q GA
> Lisa: I'm doing great, thanks. I was calling to ask if you'd like to come to a party at my house next Saturday around 8. GA
> Bob: That sounds wonderful. I'll be there for sure. GA
> Lisa: Great. C U then. Take care. Bye. GA SK
> Bob: Bye. SK SK

Directory Assistance

When you use a TTY, you won't be able to find a number by dialing 411 like you did when you used the phone in the conventional way. Information operators don't have TTYs, and relay services can't call 411 for you. There are several options, however, so find out what's avaluable. One alternative is to call AT&T's

Operator Services for the Deaf (OSD) at (800) 855-1155 (TTY) and give the operator the name and location of the business or person you want to call. OSD will then give you the number you need. The call is free, but you may be charged for the service itself.

Answering Machines

Suppose you know you won't be in, but don't want to miss an important phone message. Presto: the answering machine. A number of TTYs have built-in answering machines, which generally take only TTY messages, and many standard answering machines won't recognize a TTY call and will hang up on it. Just like telephones that can meet the needs of both deaf and hearing people, though, there are answering machines that accept either voice or TTY messages. You should expect to pay somewhere between $150 and $275 for one.

If you're in the market for a TTY/Voice answering machine, you'll want to check into the machine's message tapes. Is the outgoing message tape long enough to accommodate both the voice and TTY messages you'd like to leave? How about incoming messages — does the machine accept only messages up to a certain length, or can it record ones of any duration?

Cellular Telephones and TTY's

In the last ten or fifteen years wireless and cellular phones, which can be used without being attached to a stationary telephone jack, have become extremely popular. In fact, it's becoming more and more difficult to find someone who doesn't use one or both.

Unfortunately, deaf people have generally been unable to use both wireless and cellular phones because they weren't designed to work with a TTY. The Federal Communications Commission (FCC), which oversees telephone use in America, established June 30, 2002 as the date for digital wireless phone service to be TTY-compatible, and the major telephone companies all claim to be in compliance now. Does that mean deaf people can start using a TTY with a wireless phone? Probably not. The necessary changes have been made by providers of telephone service, but the equipment needed to take advantage of these switches isn't readily available as of this writing. That may change by the time you read this, but I'd suggest you do some checking with the FCC and the telephone provider of your choice to get the details you need before you try to use your TTY with a cellular, wireless, or specialty phone.

Another concern for deaf people who use cellular phones is that they aren't able to place an emergency call with them. Fortunately, we're seeing some important changes on that front. In West Midlands, England, for example, people with a hearing loss can report emergencies using Short Message Service, which is usually abbreviated as SMS. Limited to 160 characters (about 20 words), SMS — which is extremely popular in Europe — began in the summer of 2002. The hope is that the program will spread to police forces across Britain, and become standard in many places around the world.

Telephone Relay Services (TRS)

What are They? What are the Different Types of TRS Calls?

Until federal law mandated the establishment of a Telephone Relay Service (TRS) in every state a few years ago, TTY users could generally only communicate by telephone with others who also had a TTY, or with hearing individuals with the help of a hearing friend, business associate, or family member. Things have changed dramatically since then, however, thanks to TRS's. There are several different types of TRS calls. Following is a list of what's presently available, and a short description of each type.

Text to Voice

In this type of call the TTY user types into his or her TTY whatever he or she wants to say. The TRS's Communication Assistant (CA) then uses his or her voice to relay the typed information to the hearing person on the other end of the line.

Voice Carry-over

Late-deafened people with good speaking voices can make a voice carry-over (VCO) call when they use a TRS. This option, offered by every TRS, allows a deaf person to use his or her own voice to talk directly with the person on the other end of the line. The CA types what the hearing person says, and it appears on the deaf person's TTY, but the recipient of the call hears the voice of the deaf caller rather than that of the CA.

Hearing Carry-over:

Some users of a TRS hear well enough to use a regular phone but have a voice that's hard to understand. People in that situation can call a TRS and make what's called a Hearing Carry-Over (or HCO) call, in which an individual with a speech problem types his or her part of the conversation into a

TTY. The CA then reads the words on his or her TTY and speaks them to the called party. The caller hears the other party's replies.

Speech to Speech:

Persons with a speech disability can also use a CA who's specially trained in understanding various voice problems. The caller says something, and the CA then repeats what the caller has said in a way that makes his or her words understandable to the recipient of the call. No TTY or specialty telephone is required.

Video Relay Calls:

Late-deafened people who feel more comfortable with signed rather than spoken or text-based communication can make relay calls using Sign Language. Using a video system, they sign to a CA, who then voices what's signed for the receiving party. To make a Video Relay Call, you must have a high speed Internet connection such as DSL or Cable Modem. This service isn't required by the Federal Communications Commission, so see if it's available in your area.

Spanish Relay Calls:

Late-deafened people whose primary language is Spanish will be happy to know that telephone companies are required to provide interstate relay services in Spanish. Spanish language relay service isn't required for intrastate calls, although a number of states, particularly those with large Hispanic populations, offer it on a voluntary basis.

Voice recognition:

A late-deafened woman recently participated in a general trial of a new voice recognition phone program being sponsored by a major telephone service provider's TRS. The program isn't available in all areas, but if you have a clear voice you might find it appropriate for you. If you don't use VCO yourself, you may want to get the word about the program out to people who do. This system uses a special phone, the cost of which, after it's approved by the FCC, will be a bit more than $500. To get more information about the program, or to get into a trial yourself, you can visit the following Internet address:
http://www.ultratec.com/info/CapTel.html.

Availability and Charges

A TRS is available in each state, and operates 24 hours a day, seven days a week. There's no limit on when or how often you can use one, and a TRS allows both local and long-distance calls. Local calls are free, and long-distance ones are charged at the same rate as those made directly. Long-distance companies sometimes offer discounts on TTY calls, since they take an average of four times longer than standard voice calls. Call and get the details from your provider.

What about Privacy?

Some people are worried that the words they say in relay calls may come back to haunt them in some way. They can relax. All relay calls are strictly confidential. At most TRS centers, the CA relays the spoken and typed words of a call when they appear on a screen, and as soon as the call is completed, the screen goes blank. No record of a TRS call is kept, and CAs are trained to assure confidentiality.

Telephone Relay Services Around the Country

The following relay services are available 24 hours a day, seven days a week, 365 days a year. They're all free. "T" stands for TTY, "V" for Voice, "A" for ASC II, "B" for telebraille, "LD" for Long Distance, and "L" for Local. In a growing number of areas, simply dialing "7" or "711" will put you in touch with a TRS. Check with your chosen relay service to see if that's true for it.

T=TTY   V=Voice   A=ASCII   S=Spanish

Alabama:	(800) 548-2546 (T) (800) 548-2547 (V) (800) 548-2546 (A)	Alaska:	(800) 770-8973 (T) (800) 770-8255 (V) (800) 770-3919 (A)
Arizona:	(800) 367-8939 (T) (800) 842-4681 (V) (800) 367-8939 (A)	Arkansas:	(800) 285-1131 (T) (800) 285-1121 (V) (800) 285-1131 (A)
California:	(877) 735-2929 (T) (888) 877-5379 (V) (888) 877-5380 (A) (888) 877-5381 (S)	Colorado:	(800) 659-2656 (T) (800) 659-3656 (V) (800) 659-4656 (A)
Connecticut:	(800) 842-9710 (T) (800) 833-8134 (V) (800) 842-9710 (A)	Delaware:	(800) 232-5460 (T) (800) 232-5470 (V) (800) 232-5460 (A)
District of Columbia:	(800) 643-3768 (T) (800) 855-1000 (V) (800) 643-3768 (A)	Florida:	(800) 955-8771 (T) (800) 955-8770 (V) (800) 955-1339 (A)

Georgia:	(800) 255-0056 (T) (800) 255-0135 (V) (800) 255-0056 (A)	Hawaii:	(808) 643-8833 (T) (808) 546-2565(V) (offers "7" service)
Idaho:	(800) 377-3529 (T) (800) 377-1363 (V) (800) 377-3529 (A)	Illinois:	(800) 526-0844(T) (800) 526-0857(V) (800) 526-0844(A)
Indiana:	(800) 743-3333 (T) (800) 743-3333 (V) (800) 743-3333 (A)	Iowa:	(800) 735-2942 (T) (800) 735-2943 (V) (800) 735-2942 (A)
Kansas:	(800) 766-3777 (T) (800) 766-3777 (V) (800) 766-3777 (A)	Kentucky:	(800) 648-6056 (T) (800) 648-6057 (V) (800) 648-6058 (A)
Louisiana:	(800) 846-5277 (T) (800) 947-5277 (V) (880) 550-5277 (A)	Maine:	(800) 437-1220 (T) (800) 457-1220 (V) (800) 437-1220 (A)
Maryland:	(800) 735-2258 (T) (800) 735-2258 (V) (800) 735-2258 (A) (Offers "7" Service)	Massachusetts:	(800) 439-2370 (T) (800) 439-0183 (V) (800) 439-2370 (A)
Michigan:	(800) 649-3777 (T) (800) 649-3777 (V)	Minnesota:	(800) 627-3529 (T) (800) 627-3529 (V) (800) 627-3529 (A)
Mississippi:	(800) 582-2233 (T) (800) 855-1009 (V) (800) 855-1234 (A)	Missouri:	(800) 735-2966 (T) (800) 735-2466 (V) (800) 735-2966 (A)
Montana:	(800) 253-4091 (T) (800) 253-4093 (V) (800) 253-4091 (A)	Nebraska:	(800) 833-7352 (T) (800) 833-0920 (V) (800) 833-7352 (A)
Nevada:	(800) 326-6868 (T) (800) 326-6568 (V) (800) 326-6868 (A)	New Hampshire:	(800) 735-2964 (T) (800) 735-2964 (V) (800) 735-2964 (A)
New Jersey:	(800) 852-7899 (T) (800) 852-7897 (V) (800) 852-7899 (A)	New Mexico:	(800) 659-8331 (T) (800) 659-1779 (V) (800) 659-8331 (A)
New York:	(800) 662-1220 (T) (800) 421-1220 (V) (800) 584-2849 (A)	North Carolina:	(800) 735-2962 (T) (800) 735-8262 (V) (800) 762-2724 (A)

North Dakota:	(800) 366-6888 (T)	Ohio:	(800) 750-0750 (T)
	(800) 366-6889 (V)		(800) 750-0750 (V)
	(800) 366-6888 (A)		(800) 750-0750 (S)
			(800) 750-0750 (A)
Oklahoma:	(800) 722-0353 (T)	Oregon:	(800) 735-2900 (T)
	(800) 522-8506 (V)		(800) 735-1232 (V)
	(800) 735-3896 (S)		(800) 735-0644 (A)
	(800) 522-5065 (A)		
Pennsylvania:	(800) 654-5984 (T)	Rhode Island:	(800) 745-5555 (T)
	(800) 654-5988 (V)		(800) 745-6575 (V)
	(800) 654-5894 (A)		(800) 745-1570 (A)
South Carolina:	(800) 735-8583 (T)	South Dakota:	(800) 877-1113 (T)
	(800) 735-2905 (V)		(800) 877-1113 (V)
	(800) 735-8583 (S)		(800) 877-1113 (A)
	(800) 735-7293 (A)		
Tennessee:	(800) 848-0298 (T)	Texas:	(800) 735-2989 (T)
	(800) 848-0299 (V)		(800) 735-2988 (V)
	(800) 848-0298 (A)		(800) 735-2991 (A)
Utah:	(800) 346-4128 (T)	Vermont:	(800) 253-0191 (T)
	(800) 346-4128 (V)		(800) 253-0195 (V)
	(800) 346-4128 (A)		(800) 253-0191 (A)
	-both hearing and deaf		
Virginia:	(800) 828-1120 (T)	Washington:	(800) 833-6388 (T)
	(800) 828-1140 (V)		(800) 833-6384 (V)
	(800) 828-1120 (A)		(800) 833-6388 (A)
West Virginia:	(800) 982-8771 (T)	Wisconsin:	(800) 947-3529 (T)
	(800) 982-8772 (V)		(800) 947-6644 (V)
	(800) 982-8771 (A)		(800) 272-1773 (A)
Wyoming:	(800) 877-9965 (T)		
	(800) 877-9975 (V)		
	(800) 877-9965 (A)		
	(800) 877-9965 (S)		

In addition to the TRS's above, there are several on-line relay services that allow you to make long-distance calls by computer. In many cases they're FREE! If you have Internet access, I encourage you to check them out with a search using the term "telephone relay services" or something like that.

If you need to make a long-distance relay call and want to place it with a Relay Service other than the one that runs the TRS in your state or province, consult a publication such as <u>The Blue Book</u> by Telecommunications for the Deaf Incorporated to obtain the appropriate number. The book is also a good resource if you need a number or information that's not listed here.

Some Reminders

However you place a TRS call, it's important to keep a few things in mind:

- <u>Give the CA the name of the person you wish to speak to</u> as well as the number you want to call. If it doesn't matter who you talk to, tell the CA so.

- <u>If you want to use Voice Carryover</u>, tell the CA before he or she dials the call.

- <u>Be prepared to leave a message</u> in case the CA gets an answering machine.

- <u>Avoid long monologues.</u> When you have several questions or want to make a long statement, it helps to break them up into short bits.

- <u>Use the standard TTY abbreviations shown above, and avoid fancy punctuation</u>. If the CA isn't doing the same, ask him or her to do so. You'll save time — which can translate into big money when you make a long-distance call through a TRS.

- <u>Remember; you can't call information through a relay service</u>. Use a service specifically for deaf or hard of hearing telephone users when you need a number.

- <u>If you need the police, the fire department, or an ambulance, call 911</u>. The TRS isn't meant to serve as an emergency service. All 911 centers are required to have TTYs, and — because of pressure from advocates for the deaf and hard of hearing — are becoming more adept at using them. The reality, however, is that 911 center employees aren't always experts at handling TTY calls, and you may need to contact yours through a TRS.

LIFE AFTER DEAF

◆

Daily Life For Late-Deafened People

Is there anyone who's immune from the craziness that daily life sometimes throws at us? Nope. Acquired deafness can make being human especially challenging at times, though, so I want to suggest a few ways to help you cope more effectively with the challenges you face in day-to-day living.

<u>Driving</u>

Do you have to stop driving when you go deaf? No. Are big restrictions placed on your license after you lose your hearing? Nope. Deaf people are free to operate any kind of vehicle except a commercial one such as a truck.

Oh, you might "freak out" some people if they've never seen a deaf driver before. On a list for late-deafened people I belong to, for example, several subscribers have talked about how passengers and other drivers were sort of baffled when they saw deaf drivers signing with a passenger or looking in the mirror to read a sign or speechread someone. Being different definitely isn't against the law, though, and driving after you go deaf isn't either.

That having been said, it's important to adjust your driving habits a bit after you go deaf. To help you do that, here are a few tips:

- Mirrors, mirrors, mirrors...One late-deafened woman reported that when she went deaf she bought a siren for her car that blinks and blares when an emergency vehicle approaches. She used it for over a year and didn't see any readouts on it. Then she learned later that sirens have to be at certain frequencies for those alarms to work. So she stopped using the siren and went with a larger mirror instead.

- Another mirror tip — get a panoramic one. As the name suggests, panoramic mirrors provide a much broader view than regular types. You can find one at most auto parts stores. It will take you some time to get used to one, but with a panoramic mirror your view of what's behind you will be greatly broadened, thus making you a much safer driver.

- Speaking of mirrors…a while ago a late-deafened woman was invited to a meeting by an 85-year-old hard of hearing (hoh) friend. In the days before the meeting the deafened woman wondered how she and the hoh woman were going to communicate during the drive there. The big day arrived, the older woman showed up, and they headed off to the meeting in her car. The driver then popped up a mirror that allowed her to see both the road and her passenger's face. The late-deafened woman reports that it worked just great.

- It's also important to remain as alert as possible when you're behind the wheel. One late-deafened woman reports that a while ago she went to visit her son and was driving behind a van. She stayed well behind it because she wasn't able to see in front of it. After a while, the driver slowed down a lot and started to pull over. The woman thought he was just being nice, and passed him. Then she noticed that the cars on the other side of the road were doing the same thing as the van had done. She looked in her rear-view mirror, saw a huge fire truck bearing down on her bumper and pulled over. As I pointed out above, there are devices you can get for your car that pick up the sound of emergency vehicles, but they're of very limited usefulness. It's far wiser to remain as aware as possible of what's happening around you on the road.

Education

Education can seem out of the question when you go deaf. After all, even if you're an expert speechreader, you'll probably need to look down to take notes when you're in a classroom, and when a deaf person does that he or she will miss whatever the teacher says. But you need to keep your brain alive after your hearing goes on a permanent Spring Break. Fortunately, there are many ways to do that. If you're interested in traditional forms of schooling, the law makes it possible for you to go to a regular college with the help of a note-taker or an interpreter for the deaf. You can also attend a college for the deaf like Gallaudet University, where interaction — both in and out of the classroom — is generally based on manual rather than oral communication. Another option is to take advantage of the many correspondence courses available now, which allow you to continue your education through the mail, so you won't have to worry about your inability to hear.

If you're late-deafened, want to keep learning, and have Internet access, there are lots of on-line courses, where your lack of hearing plays absolutely no role in how much you learn. To find about courses you're interested in, do a search using the words "on-line courses" or someauch, and you'll find plenty of interesting classes.

Going back to school may help you discover a skill or interest that you never knew you had. For example, soon after I lost my hearing, I took a correspondence course in writing that allowed me to keep using my brain without relying on my hearing. While taking the course, I discovered that I love to write. Now it's a major part of my life. It allows me to keep using my brain, and to share what I've learned and think. Your discovery will most likely be different from mine, but don't be afraid to keep learning and growing just because you can't hear anymore. Do a little exploring, and you may be surprised at what you find out about yourself.

Emergencies

Although most of us don't want to think about it, there's just no escaping the reality that emergencies happen to everyone. Handling them was a major concern for late-deafened people in the past, because it was so difficult for deaf or hard of hearing persons to get information about disasters. Fortunately, that's less of a problem than it used to be. On April 14, 2000 the Federal Communications Commission (FCC) released an order adopting a rule requiring that emergency information that's provided to T.V. viewers be made accessible to persons with hearing disabilities.

What constitutes "emergency information"? Any facts about a current emergency that are intended to further the protection of life, health, safety, and property, such as critical details regarding the nature of the emergency and how to respond to it. Emergencies can be natural problems such as hurricanes, tornadoes, earthquakes, or wildfires, or man-made messes such as nuclear disasters, chemical problems, severe accidents, or acts of terrorism.

Does that mean that television information about emergencies has to be captioned? Nope. Captioning is listed as just one possible means of communicating emergency information visually. Stations can also use crawling text and/or graphics. The only requirement is that the critical information be accessible. If you'd like to learn more about what's necessary during an emergency, you can go to the web page at http://www.fcc.gov/cgb/consumerfacts/emergencyvideo.html and check out the FCC's fact sheet. If your area has experienced some kind of disaster recently and your local T.V. station didn't provide some form of visual information about it, you may want to contact the FCC at 1-888-TELL-FCC (1-888-835-5322) by TTY or 1-888-CALL-FCC (1-888-225-5322) by voice, and file a complaint. You can talk with the agency's Consumer and Mediation Specialists Monday through Friday, from 8 a.m. to 5:30 p.m. Eastern Time. When you call, be prepared to provide the following information: your name, address, and the telephone number or numbers involved with your complaint; a telephone number or e-mail address you can be reached at during the day; specific information about your complaint (the names and telephone numbers of the company representatives that you contacted are essential), the dates you spoke with them, and any other information that would help process your complaint. You should also be prepared to talk about what type of resolution you're seeking. If you have Internet access you can learn more about filing a complaint with the FCC at http://www.fcc.gov/cgb/consumerfacts/howtofile.html

Exercise

You've probably read about how exercise is good for your heart rate, blood pressure, and overall health. Learning about exercise can be challenging for late-deafened people, because they can't learn from a teacher who doesn't use sign language, listen to an audiotape on the subject, or enjoy taped music while working out. In addition, most exercise classes don't offer interpreters. Besides, just try to follow an interpreter or speechread someone and exercise at the same time and you'll know what the word "impossible" means! Fortunately, exercise isn't all that difficult for late-deafened people to master and enjoy. Here are a few things that will help.

Give your body time to get used to it.

If you're new to exercise or it's been ages since you've done any, it's a good idea to visit your doctor and see if there are any medical limitations you need to be aware of. Then start small — walking instead of jogging, for example. In many cases, particularly if you have a weight problem, your body simply isn't ready to jog or run when you start exercising. So walk instead. You'll find it a lot easier to stick with. Besides, walking is often considerably less expensive than running because it often doesn't require the specific footwear usually needed for jogging.

Don't worry that walking instead of running won't be helpful enough, though. A recent study found that women who walked briskly for two-and-a-half hours a week enjoyed the same level of protection from illness as women who did more strenuous exercises for the same amount of time.

Make new friends and re-connect with old ones

It can be difficult to create and maintain friendships after going deaf. Fortunately, it's not hard for late-deafened people to find what I call an "exercise buddy" to work out with, and getting one may help you enhance an existing friendship or create a new one.

What's an "exercise buddy?" Someone to work out with and share exercise triumphs and woes with. Exercising with a partner provides the incentive and motivation you may need to develop and stick with an exercise plan, and can help you make a new friend who shares an interest with you.

It's a good idea to find an exercise buddy who's at or near your fitness level and has exercise goals that are similar to yours. That way you can help each other. Set some groundrules too. Agree on a time to work out, and establish a procedure to follow in case one of you has to cancel a scheduled session.

Most important, exercise buddies should be supportive and positive. Encourage each other whenever necessary, especially during hard times, and provide the motivation both of you need.

There's no rule that says you can't have more than one exercise buddy, or that all of them have to be human either. Why not have several and/or take Fido out for a daily walk?

Exercise for couples

If you're married or in a long-term relationship, it's a good idea to encourage your spouse or significant other to work out with you and make him or her one of your exercise buddies. Research has shown that married couples who join a supervised fitness program together are much less likely to drop out than single people or members of a couple who join an exercise program by themselves. Besides, exercising together gives couples something to talk about. If you're not married, find a relative or friend who's willing to team up with you. That will make it a lot easier for you to develop and hang onto your enthusiasm for exercising, and will allow you to maintain long-term friendships and develop new ones.

Faith

It can be a real challenge to hang onto religious faith after you go deaf. If you go to church after you lose your hearing, you obviously won't be able to hear the pastor speak, or appreciate (or grieve over, as is often the case!) the choir's singing. Churches are exempt from the Americans with Disabilities Act, so you can't look to yours for help based on it. There are some things you can do to get more from a service, though. You'll also find that churches' leaders are usually happy to help however they can. They generally just don't know a lot about deafness, and need you to suggest things they can do to make worshipping as satisfying as possible for you. To help you do that, here are a few recommendations:

- Make friends with other members of your parish, as well as your priest, reverend, rabbi, or pastor. Let the church's leaders see that your hearing loss doesn't have to prevent you from helping the church or synagogue in ways that are appropriate for your skills and experience.

- Churches, temples, and mosques are usually on a tight budget, so they often can't afford to do everything you'd like them to. Therefore, it's a good idea to take advantage of the many free or low-cost benefits modern technology provides. For example, have copies of homilies e-mailed to you whenever possible. That's a lot less expensive than CART, so it's real music to the ears of cash-strapped religious institutions.

- If you still have some residual hearing left, and know of other parishioners who are hard of hearing, suggest that your church, mosque, or temple be wired for FM devices. Chances are quite good that your religious institution's staff simply doesn't know much about that sort of thing, and will welcome your input.

- Focus on your abilities rather than your disability. For example, a while ago I put together an insert for my church's bulletin. It was a great way for me to provide some much-needed free help for my church, and my deafness didn't affect my ability to do so. Best of all, it made me feel like I was really part of the church's family.

Humor

Many people who go deaf feel like humor and laughter are sort of out of the question once their hearing call it quits. They're not. While it's true that deafness imposes some very real limits on what late-deafened people can laugh at because their loss prevents them from hearing what others say, I'm happy to report that "laugh after deaf" is very real.

Why is laughter so important? Because it's good for both the body and the spirit. If you'd like to learn about how and why that's true, there are a couple of books you'll want to check out. The first is <u>Anatomy of an Illness as Perceived by the Patient</u> by Norman Cousins. The author, who was editor of the magazine *Saturday Review* for several years, recovered from a supposedly fatal illness called Amyotrophic Lateral Sclerosis (better known as ALS or Lou Gehrig's Disease in honor of the famed baseball player who died from it) by following a program that included large doses of Vitamin C and plenty of laughter. The book details the many benefits laughter provided the author in his trip to recovery, and extols the physical benefits of laughter, which he likens to "jogging internally without having to go outdoors." The physical benefits of laughter include: strengthening the immune system, stimulating the circulation, assisting the lungs and respiratory system, increasing the number of T-cells that have helper/receptors, lowering serum cholesterol levels, reducing stress hormones, relaxing muscles, boosting the number and activity of natural killer cells, providing an aerobic workout, and reducing pain.

Laughter provides a lot more than physical pluses though. In fact, I could probably write an entire book about the emotional benefits laughing and smiling provide. Thankfully, someone has done exactly that. If you're in the mood for an encouraging, entertaining, and intelligent look at the spiritual advantages of laughter, check out <u>The Healing Power of Humor</u> by Allen Klein, which includes a foreword by the well-known physician O. Carl Simonton that speaks of the "profound power of laughter, humor, and play." The mental benefits of laughter include: the power to cope, emotional strength, and the broadening of one's perspective.

Since going deaf, I've been privileged to "hear" some hysterical (and true!) hearing-related stories from late-deafened people. I don't want to be greedy, so here's my favorite. You can file it under "revenge is sweet."

◆   ◆   ◆

One evening a telemarketer called the home of a late-deafened man (at dinner time of course!). His college-age hearing son answered, and the caller said "This is the Acme Carpet Cleaning Company. May I speak to Mr. Smith please?" The son replied that his father was deaf and offered to take a message. The caller said something like "No, that's O.K., I'll call back later." The son replied that his father would still be deaf later and said he'd be happy to take a message and pass it on to his dad. Then the caller came out with the following inanity: "Well, that's O.K. Deaf people don't need their carpets cleaned anyway." The son questioned that ridiculous statement, and the caller responded by hanging up.

The teen was angered, and grabbed the phone book to get the company's number. He then phoned the company, and his call was answered by the same person who'd just hung up on him. "May I speak with the owner or manager, please?" the son asked. "Sorry," came the reply. "he's not in. May I take a message?" "Yes," the son said. "I wish to speak with him regarding his telephone sales program." "Oh," the voice on the other end of the line replied "We have no phone sales program." "Fine," the boy said. "Please give me the company's mailing address." "Well, I don't know what it is," the man answered, and hung up abruptly.

The son checked the phone book, though, and easily found the company's address. So he wrote a short letter to the owner explaining what had happened and complaining about the caller. Then he sent it off. A couple evenings later, the owner called the late-deafened man's house, and the son answered. The owner claimed that the original caller was just a temporary worker who was no longer with the company. He then said "But we'd still like to clean your carpets. And we'll give you a discount." The son's reply?: "Well thanks. That's very nice of you. But deaf people don't need their carpets cleaned." Click.

Medicine

Although late-deafened people face many challenges in life, one of the most significant is that of finding and benefiting from good medical care. Although the Americans with Disabilities Act protects the rights of disabled individuals who already have a doctor, many physicians simply refuse to accept new patients who have a disability. That doesn't happen all the time, of course — there are many M.D.'s who welcome new patients of any kind — but you shouldn't be surprised if being deaf makes it difficult for you to find good medical care. In addition, even though your M.D. may provide an interpreter for an appointment or (gulp!) surgery, your signing skills may be too limited for you to benefit significantly from one. So I'd like to make some suggestions for enjoying better health and getting more satisfying results from trips to your doctor.

- The most important step, of course, is to become less dependent on physicians. This isn't to say that doctors aren't important, and you should certainly avail yourself of all the help they can provide. As physician and best-selling author Bernie Siegel once joked, however, some patients and doctors seem to think that "M.D." stands for "Medical Deity." As a result, the patient loses — or hands over, really — his or her autonomy. Doctors can help patients find a cause for a medical problem they're having, but ultimately, only you know what's right for you. You can't always rely on a medical professional to understand what's right for you, and you shouldn't expect that of him or her.

- Eat right. Although there are all sorts of healthy foods now, the percentage of obese people in America is at an all-time high. Why? Part of the problem is fat-free foods. Well, not the foods themselves, but the folks who eat lots and lots of them figuring that if a food is fat-free they can eat as much of it as they want. So they eat a lot and end up consuming considerably more calories than they burn. As a result, they gain weight, and by doing that increase their cholesterol level. That, in turn, raises their risk of heart attack, stroke, and life-threatening illnesses.

- Another section of this chapter looks at sleep, so I won't talk about it in depth here. I just want to remind you to get to bed at a reasonable hour so you can give your body a chance to rest up after all the work involved in being human. Sometimes in the quest to get ahead, we end up sacrificing sleep, and hence, our health. That can be particularly true for the late-deafened, because many things we do take longer than when we could hear. So we sleep less than we should.

Read — and Keep Your Brain Alive

Reading is a wonderful way for late-deafened people to gather information or simply be entertained. It allows them to be sure of something, unlike speechreading or sign language. Doing lots of reading is also good for our health. A study done not too long ago found that people who regularly engaged in various intellectual activities such as reading books, magazines, and newspapers were significantly less likely to develop Alzheimer's disease than individuals who didn't. Benefits didn't come just from reading, of course — playing games such as checkers and going to museums were also found to be helpful. It was using the mind that was beneficial.

Keeping your brain alive by doing things like reading can also help you stay young. While there's no surefire way to prevent diseases that weaken the mind, more and more research suggests that engaging in mentally challenging activities like reading can help us stay physically healthy.

Reading can also be a great tool for sharing humor. One of the first parts of the newspaper that I read every morning (and sometimes it's the *only* part!) is the comics page, because I can enjoy the visual pleasure the comics provide and be sure of what's said in them. Besides, comic strips are often really funny — an important consideration for a guy who put together a collection of humor called He Who Laughs Lasts in 2001.

Reunions and Parties

Maybe I'm strange (well, I know I am!) but there are few things that make me as anxious as a family reunion or party. Although I'm usually friends with most of the people who attend the ones I go to, I'm also almost always the only deaf person there. Virtually no one else knows any sign language, and even when there are a few signers present, most of them aren't willing to slow down their signing enough to have a real conversation with a thoroughly mediocre signer like me. So we end up talking briefly about topics like the weather or whatever, and have a truly forgettable conversation.

In the summer of 2002, I took a trip to Connecticut to see some family members and friends. Part of me was really excited about the visit in the weeks before I headed north, but there was another side of me that didn't look forward to it at all because of the communication problems that always arise when I'm with family members and hearing friends I've known for ages. Fortunately, there are a few things late-deafened people can do to maximize their enjoyment and minimize their stress when it comes to things like visits, reunions, and parties.

- Before you go see family and friends, contact them individually and let them know what you want to do to maximize interaction with them. Rather than focusing on all the things they usually *don't* do when they communicate with you, emphasize what they *can* do. Stay as positive as possible. People respond much more affirmatively to "yes" than "no" messages, so when you talk with others about communicating with you try to accentuate the positive elements and steer clear of the negative ones.

- Remember that when you go to a party or other gathering you don't have to stay for the whole thing. Why not just put in an appearance, and tell the people you see there that you'll talk with them in depth later? Parties can be lots of fun, but if you're anything like me you probably find it much more satisfying to communicate with people in one-on-one situations or in small groups.

- Don't forget, either, that the fun of a party or gathering isn't solely a product of the ability to hear. For example, when a neighbor's daughter had her first birthday party recently, and I was the only deaf person in attendance, I had a great time watching her blow out the single candle on her birthday cake and seeing the obvious glee she felt in unwrapping the presents she got. I sure didn't need any hearing to do either.

- You don't have to be "on" the whole time you're at a party or reunion. There's nothing wrong with taking a break, having a drink, resting, or being alone. After you've kicked back a bit, gather yourself up again and rejoin the festivities.

Pets

In the assistive devices chapter, I talked about the positive role hearing dogs often play in the lives of many late-deafened people. You might want to think about getting one for yourself. If you choose not to, you could consider getting some other kind of four-legged friend. A recent study found that individuals who owned a cat or dog had significantly lower blood pressure and stress levels than those who didn't.

Led by Dr. Karen Allen of the State University of New York, the study involved 240 married couples, half of whom owned a cat or dog, and half who didn't. Researchers investigated the effects of spouses, pets, and close friends (for non-pet owners) on the participants' responses to various stressful stimuli, including immersing a hand in ice water for two minutes, and performing mental arithmetic. All the participants had normal blood pressure.

The findings? Whether active or at rest, participants who owned pets had considerably lower heart rates and blood pressure levels than those who didn't. The study also found that pet owners were most calm when their cats or dogs were present, whereas participants who didn't have a cat or dog were at their calmest when they were alone. Pet owners also showed a considerably smaller change in their heart rate and blood pressure when they did the hands-in-cold-water test.

Why were pet-owners more relaxed than those who didn't have a cat or dog? Perhaps, as Allen suggested, pet owners view their furry friends as totally non-judgmental and accepting, so they're not afraid to try something for fear of failing at it. It isn't clear if owning pets directly caused the lower stress and blood-pressure levels, but as Dr. Allen said "we do encourage people who like animals and have time for them to consider the potential advantage of the healthy pleasure of their company."

Relaxation

Speaking of being more relaxed...

Did you know that the word "relax" comes from the Latin term "relaxare," which means "to loosen"? That's exactly what relaxing is — a loosening. When you relax, you loosen life's grip on you and let go of unwanted tension and anxiety. Unfortunately, late-deafened people often find it hard to relax, especially after a day, week, month, or years of not being able to hear what's said to them or the sounds in the world. Fortunately, there's an easy solution to the problem.

As I pointed out earlier in the chapter about psychology, a great way to relax is to pay close attention to your breathing. Probably the best way to do that is to meditate. Check out that chapter for instructions on how to do that. There are also all sorts of articles and books on the subject of meditation, and because reading doesn't require hearing, learning how to meditate via reading is easy for late-deafened people. Give it a try, and you'll probably be amazed by the change in you.

Sleep

You can't really talk about relaxation without discussing sleep. After all, sleep is the most effective form of relaxation there is. Many of us are taught as children that humans need six to eight hours of sleep a day, but it can be difficult to get that much as adults because of work commitments, social obligations, and a desire to spend time with friends and family. As I've said before, doing things when your ears no longer work can take markedly longer than it used to, and many late-deafened people, as a result, try to get by with less than the recommended amount of sleep. We promise ourselves that we'll catch up on the weekend or whenever, but when they come, we often have trouble drifting off. So I want to give you some practical suggestions that will make it easier for you to sleep.

- Spend more time with others. It can be difficult to spend quality time with people after you go deaf, but a recent study shows how important that is. It found that those who feel lonely may have more trouble sleeping at night than those who spend lots of time with friends and family. Besides, as the free e-mail service "RealAge Tip of the Day" reports, having a strong support network can make your "RealAge" up to three-and-a-half years younger than the calendar says you are.

- Is your bed comfortable, and not too soft or too hard? Check your mattress a couple times a year for wear and tear, and replace it immediately if it's too hard, too soft, or lumpy. What about your pillow? Is it right for you, or do you need a new one?

- Are aches or pains keeping you awake? Get yourself to a doctor.

- Are you a caffeine "junkie"? While many people rely on coffee to help them get started in the morning, you should see if it's keeping you awake when you'd rather be asleep (work excluded, of course!). If that's the case, you might want to switch to decaf, or drink only decaffeinated beverages a few hours before you hit the sack. If you're wary of sleeping pills, and are looking for some non-prescription help nodding off, you might want to try the supplement Valerian Root. Several people I know use it, and report it's really helped them fall asleep. It's also considerably less expensive than prescription and over-the-counter drugs that help people sleep.

- A big obstacle to sleep for many people is a mind that stays in overdrive when it's time for sleep. If that's a problem for you, try a little gentle stretching or relaxing breathing just before you hit the hay. That should help you calm yourself and avoid the "wandering-mind" syndrome.

- Another breathing tip…If falling asleep when you first go to bed or after getting up in the middle of the night is a problem for you, here's a suggestion. Instead of letting your mind wander after you lie down — worrying about something you have to do tomorrow, for instance — do a little "neo-meditating" and focus on just one thing: your breathing. Breathe deeply and slowly, and pay close attention to that. If your mind wanders, don't give yourself a hard time. Just go back to breathing deeply and focusing on it. You'll usually fall asleep very quickly.

Small Pleasures

My wife and I live in a townhouse in the Maryland suburbs of D.eaf C.ity. Many times, a townhouse is the first house newlyweds buy, and they later move to a bigger place when they have kids and/or start making more money. Older people sometimes buy townhouses after their kids have moved away. Townhouses — whether purchased by newlyweds or older couples — are often a short-term housing choice.

By contrast, Mary and I have lived in our townhouse for more than a decade. We don't have any plans to move any time soon, either. For one thing, we really don't need the extra space a bigger house would provide. For another, we really love the area we live in.

There's another reason for our desire to stay put, though. You see, Mary's turned our backyard into sort of a green heaven. There aren't just flowers all over the place, but the entire backyard is covered with shrubs and exotic plants. The number of hours and amount of effort Mary's put into creating and maintaining our backyard paradise is truly impressive — and the joy it brings us isn't something either of us wants to give up.

While I dearly love all the greenery we have outside our house, I'm even happier about something else — that Mary has found so much joy in such a simple pleasure. Do you have one that makes you especially happy? Then do it. Yes, being late-deafened prevents us from doing certain things that we might want to do (I've never heard of a deaf rock star, for instance!), but there's nothing that says we can't take great pleasure in the things we *can* do. I said before that I don't particularly agree with the statement that "deaf people can do anything but hear," but there's no reason that our inability to hear should prevent us from taking great pleasure in all the small things we're able to do after our ears stop working.

Technology

Over the past few years technology has really taken off, making life easier and more interesting for virtually everyone. Late-deafened people have benefited considerably from the boom in technology, especially the growing use of computers, because they allow people to do so many things that would have been difficult or impossible in the past because of their inability to hear.

A late-deafened friend who's in his 50's reports that while he's generally pretty immune to amazement he's absolutely in awe of today's technology. His family didn't even have a black and white television when he was a baby, and today he can't imagine his life without his computer, e-mail, and access to the Internet. Aside from using his computer to stay in touch with family and friends, the volunteer work he does is conducted via the Internet. His rheumatologist even e-mails him to schedule some of his appointments. Instant access to huge amounts of information on the Web is truly wonderful to him too. As he puts it, "this explosion of technology is an absolute life-changer!"

You can use the Internet to do virtually anything now — even to take a hearing test. The test results are greatly influenced by the quality of the sound card and speakers on your computer, of course, but the site the test is on (http://www.freehearingtest.com/) is definitely worth a visit.

Television and Movies

A while ago I read a quotation that said "Theater is art; cinema is imagination; television is furniture." Besides loving the praise of theater (I was very involved in it before I went deaf) and laughing hysterically at the joke about television being furniture, I also got to thinking about how important T.V. can be in our culture. It may be "furniture," but television is a major source of entertainment and information for many people, and there's no need to do without it after you go deaf. Some television directories indicate captioned programs by including "CC" next to the listing for them. An increased number of televised advertisements are also captioned. Many late-deafened people don't buy items on the basis of television advertisements for them, but captioned commercials have allowed deafened consumers to feel like they're a significant part of the buying public.

If you've never seen a captioned program or advertisement, it's easy to adjust your television to show captions. If you don't have a television that allows you to do that, corral a family member or friend whose T.V. can display captions. Most people will be happy to let you see what they look like. You can also head to a store that sells television sets, and explain to the salesperson that you'd like to see the closed captioning on one. He or she will almost always be happy to help you.

Emergency announcements, unfortunately, still often aren't captioned. For example, many of the television reports about the snipers who terrorized the D. C. area in the Fall of 2002 offered no captions. The good news, though, is that the Northern Virginia Resource Center for Deaf and Hard of Hearing Persons, led by Executive Director Cheryl Heppner (a former ALDA president), formally complained about that. The Federal Communications Commission is investigating the issue as of this writing.

Some deafened people are more comfortable than others with captions. You often have to read them very quickly in order to take in an entire caption before it's replaced with the next one, and it can be difficult to read one completely while keeping up with the non-verbal action on the screen. So you may need to practice a little when you start out.

We all need something beyond television at times, of course, and I'm happy to report that movies — both at home and beyond — are a great entertainment option for late-deafened people. The world of movie-going is changing constantly, but the following will give you a good idea of what's available now and how best take advantage of it.

Let's start with movie-watching at home. If you decide to rent or buy a videotape or a DVD of a film, it's important to make sure it contains a symbol showing it's captioned (usually the letters "CC" surrounded by the image of a television) before you give up any of your hard-earned cash. DVD's sometimes don't have the "CC" symbol on them, but they're usually captioned, although if you want assurance, you can always ask a sales clerk. The vast majority of films recorded these days are captioned, but some documentaries and many older movies that are re-recorded aren't. Video and DVD rental stores often provide a catalogue that identifies which of their films are captioned, though, and it's a good idea to consult one of those before renting or buying a videotape or disk if you're uncertain.

If you want to head out and see a movie in a theater, you'll be happy to know that there's an increasing number of showings of open-captioned films. You can contact movie theaters directly to see when they're offering captioned showings of films or talk with deaf friends to find out what's available in your area. I've been to several open-captioned showings in the past few years, and can attest that there's a tremendous difference between seeing a film on a movie screen and watching a DVD or videocassette on your television.

A growing number of theaters are also experimenting with a relatively new kind of captioning. Rather than appearing as text on the top or bottom of the theater's screen, dialogue in these showings appears as captions that show up on a screen at the back of the seat in front of selected ones. You can do a little homework and learn when and where this kind of showing is available in your area.

Another good option for late-deafened movie-goers is a public showing of a subtitled foreign film, where the dialogue appears in print at the bottom of the screen. Several years ago my wife and I went to a subtitled showing of the Italian film *Life is Beautiful,* and to this day it's one of my favorite films, which I'm sure has a lot to do with the fact that I saw it in a movie theater rather than on a television with a VCR or DVD player.

Time — How Not to Sweat it

Do you feel harried before you run off to work, church, your kid's soccer match, a meeting, or whatever because there's still a lot to do? Join the crowd! Everyone feels rushed at times. That can be a big problem for late-deafened people, especially those who are also physically disabled, because after their losses almost everything they do takes longer than it used to. In time, feeling hurried and harried becomes sort of a regular part of post-deafness life, and as a result it serves as yet another source of stress for us.

Fortunately, there's an easy solution to the problem: giving yourself an extra ten minutes to get ready before you head out the door. Ten minutes might not seem like a whole lot of time, but you'll be amazed how much easier it makes your life if you give yourself that much more time to get ready for something. Do it and you'll find how much less stress you feel, and how much more enjoyable life is.

It can be difficult to make a change in our lifestyles, so if the idea of getting up a bit earlier in the morning than you used to is daunting, you may want to go to bed a few minutes earlier than you did in the past. That way, getting up a bit earlier won't be too hard. In time, the change will become habit, and you'll find that the benefits of rising a few minutes earlier than you used to far outweigh the advantages of getting a little extra shut-eye. Besides the obvious benefit of eliminating the need to run around like mad before you head out the door, getting up a few minutes earlier than you used to will also allow you to enjoy events more after you arrive at them — because you'll feel less stressed out.

Travel

Traveling after you go deaf can be a real challenge. Late-deafened people who take a trip won't hear instructions and information provided by pilots, stewardesses, ship captains, and the like. There's great potential for travel-related stress in deafened people. That's simply an obstacle to be overcome, though, and Joan Cassidy, a late-deafened woman who frequently takes cruises with her hearing husband Neil, offers some helpful tips for people with imperfect or non-existent hearing who want to hit the road. Joan's suggestions are based on her extensive experiences with cruises, but many of them apply to virtually any kind of traveling.

Joan's Cruise Tips (a.k.a. "Never Give Up the Ship!")

My husband Neil and I have taken 18 cruises, most of them on Princess®. It's the most relaxing way to travel, especially for someone with a severe hearing loss. We spend as little money as possible on the trip itself but always tip at least the suggested amount. I also write a thank-you note after we return, naming the people who helped make it a great voyage. I make a lot of special requests, but Princess treats me (okay, I'll say it) like a princess, and always makes us feel welcome.

Federal courts have ruled that the ADA applies to foreign flagged cruise ships if they sail in U.S. waters or dock at a U.S. port, and of course they're not going to tear out the listening system, TTYs, or other assistive equipment after the ship sails away from the US. In the last few years the major cruise lines have started to do a lot more to help passengers with hearing loss, but they usually don't tell us what they have. They've spent millions making their ships accessible to passengers with disabilities, though, and now it's up to us to ask for the assistance we need.

Most ships can provide a TTY, closed-captioned TV, a flashing light for the doorbell, and a visual alarm system. Newer ships have assistive listening systems in the show lounges. If you ask in advance, some cruise lines will arrange to have a sign language interpreter on board for the shows and tours. Your service dog can travel with you, but you must notify the cruise line in advance and provide written proof that your dog is a certified service animal. Some countries won't allow the dog on shore, so check in advance. There are also several specific steps you should take, whether you use a service dog or not:

1. Do it yourself. You're the expert, and you know what you need, so you should do the work. Don't leave it to your travel agent. E-mail, write, or call the cruise line, ask for Special Services, and explain in detail exactly what you need and why. Get something in writing (letter or e-mail) listing what the ship will have available and take the letter with you.

2. Don't give up easily. Employees at cruise headquarters often know little about hearing access and will just say they have nothing available, so ask to speak to someone higher up. This applies on the ship too, because you may be the first passenger to ask for a TTY, flashing light for the doorbell, or captioned TV. The equipment is probably easily available and just locked away in a cupboard somewhere.

3. People make the difference. Even if things go wrong and there is no assistive equipment on board, you can still have a good cruise. The Maitre d' can get you a table in the quietest part of the dining room with a waiter or waitress who's easy to understand. Ask for a table for two if that will make your meals more relaxing. The Tour Desk staff can reserve a seat near the front of the tour bus for you so you can speechread the guide, and may be able to provide written information about the tour. The Cruise Director can reserve seats up front in the show lounge and try to get you written scripts of lectures, though some presenters may refuse to hand over their notes. The Purser's Desk can track down a TV with captions and possibly a VCR and some captioned videos. I've ended up with the TV or VCR from the gym or officers'

mess and videos borrowed from the crew. One ship arranged for a listening system to be flown to the next port the ship was stopping at. We've been invited onto the bridge so I could speechread the park guide in Glacier Bay and get a great view while going through the Panama Canal. SO SPEAK UP! Cruise lines want you to be happy, but their employees can't read your mind.

Remember:

- Do it yourself. You're the expert.

- Don't take "no" for an answer until you get it from the CEO of the cruise line. If that happens, take your business elsewhere and find a cruise line that has what you need.

- Never give up. There is always something that can make the situation better. Cruise ships are full of people who want you to enjoy your trip.

- If all fails, ask in writing for a refund, giving details of what went wrong. This applies to everyone, deaf or hearing.

- Buy travel insurance — illness, accidents, or cancellations can happen to anyone.

Have fun!

◆   ◆   ◆

Walking Off Stress

The chapter about the psychology of late-deafness talked about the issue of stress, and as anyone who's late-deafened can tell you, there are times when not being able to hear really makes you want to scream. It's a good idea, though, to get rid of stress whenever possible. In addition to causing mental pain, stress is also bad for your body. It increases both your heart rate and blood pressure, and recent studies have shown that frequent exposure to stress hormones may also weaken your memory considerably.

Fortunately, there's a simple step you can take to keep stress to a minimum: daily walks. I know what you're thinking: "Who has time for regular walks?" Good news! Research has found that three 10-minute walks taken at different times during the day — maybe one before work, a second at lunch time, and a third after dinner — are as effective at preventing or limiting stress as a single 30-minute constitutional. Although the thought of exercise can be sort of stressful in and of itself, the fact is that it's actually a good way to counteract the anxious moods we all have at times.

Another benefit: walking can improve circulation — which, in turn, may help you feel more alert, and decrease blood levels of stress hormones. Recent studies have also shown that regular exercise can help alleviate the feelings of mild depression almost all of us have at times, and do it as effectively as prescription medications.

Walking's also a good way to save money — a huge stress-reliever in and of itself. The footwear required for certain sports can be quite specific and expensive. For example, just check out the prices of the sneakers needed for running or basketball. Walking, by contrast, doesn't require any special footwear — plain old sneakers are fine. Several late-deafened people I know walk extensively, and they save the money they'd have to spend for the special footwork required for other forms of exercise and use it for more "exciting" things like paying for car repairs or their kids' college expenses.

Work

The issue of deafened people at work easily merits an entire book, and I hope someone will write one soon. Until that happens, here are some ideas you can use to help make your experiences on the job as positive as possible. As with all suggestions in this book, the following should be adapted to fit your particular needs and interests.

- Be sure that the workplace is adequately lighted. That's especially true of rooms used for meetings or training.
- An employer should provide necessary visual alerting devices.
- If environmental noise contributes to communication difficulties, the affected worker should be put in a quieter place.
- The work station/office should be arranged so that the worker can easily see someone entering.
- Assistive listening devices should be in place.
- Oral or sign-language interpreters should be available when needed.
- Note takers should be used in meetings and group discussions.

- Co-workers and bosses should be politely made aware of personal habits that can interfere with comfortable speechreading, such as chewing gum or eating while talking, or not facing a deaf employee when speaking to him or her.

- Employees and supervisors should use e-mail, fax machines, and computer note-taking for intra-and inter-office communication whenever possible.

- Videotaped training materials should be captioned.

- Real-time captioning should be used for meetings and training sessions.

Closely related to the issue of work is volunteering. One of my most satisfying experiences after going deaf was volunteering at Gallaudet University's National Information Center on Deafness, where I won the university's "Volunteer Rookie of the Year" award for the 1992–93 academic year and became the NICD's resident "expert" on acquired deafness. Volunteering might be right for you too. Is there a church, school, or charitable organization near you that can benefit from what you have to offer? Grab the phone book or talk to a friend, and you might be surprised to learn what's out there.

◆   ◆   ◆

There you have it! Following the suggestions above may leave you repeating the title of that marvelous film — "It's a Wonderful Life."

HEARING AIDS

An Overview

People who become hard of hearing are often traumatized by that, but this may just be the best time yet to have less-than-perfect hearing. That's not because of any great medical advances in the field of hearing loss — after all, doctors are still mystified as to what causes certain people to lose some or all of their hearing, and there are no cures for hearing loss except the ones offered by quacks and money-hungry individuals. Instead, it's because of all the different kinds of hearing aids that are available now. Hearing aids are a very personal matter, and people who are thinking of getting them are advised to confer with a professional to learn what they need to know. Hearing aids aren't of any use to individuals who are totally deaf, but deafened people with residual hearing who have hearing aids often speak very highly of them.

It's also important for people who get hearing aids to have realistic expectations for them. Hearing aids don't make you a "hearie" again. They simply amplify the sounds you receive. Even the most powerful hearing aids might not be strong enough for your particular needs. You'll have to decide — with help from your audiologist or hearing aid specialist — if getting them is right for you. That having been said, though, here are some ideas to help you make your way through what might seem like the perplexing jungle of hearing aids.

If you feel a bit baffled by all the technological advances over the past several years, you can relax when it comes to hearing aids. While many different kinds of hearing aids are available now, and there's been lots of progress in the field over the years, there's not much mystery about what hearing aids do. They simply amplify the sounds you hear, and may allow you to use the telephone without a TTY or watch television without a decoder. If you're thinking that you shouldn't bother with the expense or inconvenience of hearing aids because you hear almost nothing now, it might help to remember that hearing aids can improve your speechreading ability markedly or help you understand sign language better because they add auditory input to the visual clues you receive.

Resistance

Getting your first hearing aids is a big step, and your resistance to wearing them in public may interfere with the purchase and successful use of them. When a test in 1987 indicated I would need to wear hearing aids, for example, I nodded politely to the PhD who conducted the exam and gave me the news, walked calmly to the parking lot, and started to scream as soon as I reached the safety of my car. I was only 26! How could I possibly sustain the image I had so carefully cultivated of an active, energetic young man if I had to wear hearing aids?

I was about to learn one of the most important lessons of hearing loss — that acknowledging that we need hearing aids to help us hear better can be difficult. We want to be perfect, and — at least when we're younger — we like to think of ourselves as indestructible. Yet wearing hearing aids says we're not flawless, and when we need to wear them after years of normal hearing, we're reminded that we're not indestructible either. We often greet the prospect of wearing our first hearing aids by forgetting the adage that's become so popular with people in hearing-related professions: "Your hearing aids are far less conspicuous than your hearing loss."

Testing, Testing…

One of the first things you'll want to do after you become concerned about your hearing is to get it thoroughly evaluated by an audiologist, otolaryngologist (an Ear, Nose, and Throat specialist, often called an ENT), or hearing aid dispenser. The test will tell you if hearing aids can help you, and during your visit you'll also learn what advantages different types of aids offer.

Hearing tests vary, but they generally work like this:

- You enter a room with thick padding. You wear a pair of headphones, and the audiologist, otolaryngologist, or hearing aid dispenser sits outside the room and watches you through a small window. You can hear his or her voice through the headphones.

- He or she uses a machine that produces sounds at different volumes and frequencies that can be heard through the headphones. You'll raise your hand or push a button when these sounds are just loud enough for you to hear them. The left and right ears are tested separately, and the tester generally starts with higher frequencies and moves on to lower ones. Physicists learn early in their training that frequency is a measure of the number of sine waves per second, but for the rest of us it's probably enough to know that women and children generally have higher voices (at faster frequencies) than grown men.

- In what's usually the second half of the test, the tester will pronounce certain one- and two-syllable words for you, and ask you to repeat them (you'll be told something like "say the word 'house'"). The tester blocks your view of his or her mouth while saying the words, so you'll rely on just your hearing and not your speechreading ability to understand what's said.

The results of the test are recorded on an audiogram, which tells you what your hearing level is at various frequencies. Based on the results of these tests, the tester will determine what kind of hearing aid, if any, will help you the most.

Before you commit to a particular model, the tester may let you take a hearing aid home and try it for a day or two to get a better feeling of what it's like to wear one. During this trial period, don't expect miraculous, instantaneous results. One disabled person has pointed out that "canes help you get around easier, but they don't make your leg better," and a similar truth applies to hearing aids — they help you hear better by making sounds louder, but they don't restore any of your hearing. Most can be programmed to focus on certain frequencies, so the voices around you sound louder (which means they'll be easier to understand), but you won't hear perfectly with a hearing aid. You might also experience a corresponding increase in the volume of dishes being put away, a drip in the kitchen sink, or certain other sounds you'd probably rather do without.

It also takes time for the human body to get used to hearing aids. Studies indicate that many people experience a decline in their speech intelligibility at the end of the first 30 days of hearing aid use, but a marked increase in it after 60 to 90 days. Improvements also have been noted after three to six months of hearing aid use. So be a patient patient.

One Versus Two

Some potential hearing aid users wonder if the extra expense of buying two aids instead of one is really worth it. Without going into an extensive discussion of the one-versus-two debate, I want to point out that there are at least three reasons why a pair of hearing aids is often more beneficial than one.

First, if you have a hearing loss in both ears, wearing two aids will improve your ability to hear different sounds. With a pair of hearing aids, your brain will combine the sounds received by both ears, which will make you more sensitive to them.

Second, wearing two aids instead of one can improve your directionality — your ability to know where a particular sound is coming from. That can help your interaction with people and increase your safety.

Finally, wearing two aids instead of one can make it easier for you to listen in groups. You may not have to turn your head or ask people to speak into your "good ear."

Your First Hearing Aids

If you decide to get hearing aids, an impression will be taken with soft, spongy material for the earmold — the part of the hearing aid that goes in your ear canal. Depending on your degree of hearing loss, you will wear in-the-ear or behind-the-ear hearing aids, which both have ear-molds. Those with milder hearing losses often wear small aids that sit completely in the ear canal. Canal aids, such as those worn by former U.S. president Ronald Reagan, don't require ear-molds, and new technology is being used to produce canal aids that are small but extremely powerful. Another type of hearing aid, which was just developed recently, is the bone-anchored hearing aid. A screw is surgically implanted in the skull behind the ear, and a hearing aid is attached to it. In the past, many hard of hearing individuals used a body aid, a large (about 2" x 4") unit that was attached to a shirt, dress, or sweater. Body aids, however, are becoming increasingly rare, and hearing aid users generally opt for smaller, lighter models that either fit completely within the ear or sit behind it.

Will you need to wear your hearing aids all the time after you get your first ones? There's considerable debate about the matter of getting accustomed to hearing aids. Some hearing professionals feel that the best way to become comfortable with a hearing aid is for new users to wear it whenever they're awake. They argue that the brain and nervous system need time to adjust to the body's new hearing level, and the consistent use of new hearing aids will make that process easier, faster, and more complete. Other individuals, however, feel that people can take their time becoming accustomed to wearing aids, and that users should remove theirs whenever they feel the need to.

Cost And Financial Help

There are other obstacles besides stigma to purchasing hearing aids, especially cost. Good hearing aids aren't cheap, and we've probably all heard or read horror stories about people who've bought expensive aids only to have them malfunction or deliver less-than-wonderful results. We don't want to spend lots of money on hearing aids unless we can be sure we're looking at a worthwhile investment, and for many of us the assurance we get in the form of trial, exchange, and refund periods just isn't enough.

In truth, however, today's hearing aids usually have good warrantees and can actually cost less in real dollars than the hearing instruments of several years ago. Today's price tag often includes the cost of many benefits that were limited or unheard of in the past, such as diagnostic procedures, counseling, and aftercare services. Some hearing aid dispensers sell aids with these services, while others oppose this kind of "bundling" and sell aids independent of options like those just mentioned at a considerably lower price. You should talk with your hearing aid specialist for details and prices.

If you've decided to get hearing aids but aren't sure how you'll swing the expense, you might look to the following agencies and organizations for information or help:

The International Hearing Society (IHS): The IHS has its own toll-free National Hearing Helpline. Call (800) 521-5247 (Voice) to find out what kind of assistance is available.

American Speech-Language-Hearing Association (ASHA) : ASHA provides information about insurance coverage for hearing aids and related hearing services. Also listed in "A Resource Resource," ASHA can be reached by telephone at (800) 638-8255 (Voice/TTY), faxed at (301) 897-7348, or written to at American Speech-Language-Hearing Association, Healthcare Financing Division, 10801 Rockville Pike, Rockville, MD, 20852. You can also find all sorts of information about ASHA on the group's web page (http://www.asha.org/about/contacts.cfm).

Rehabilitation Services Administration (RSA): Contact your local RSA office, usually part of a government agency, to see what kind of assistance is available when paying for hearing aids.

U.S. Veterans Administration: Veterans of various wars can receive free hearing aids if they meet certain requirements. Contact your local Veterans Administration office for details.

Civic and Service Organizations: Your telephone directory will provide the names of organizations in your area that offer help with hearing-related expenses. Many receive donations to provide hearing aids and other assistive listening devices for people who need them. Groups that can help include:

National Easter Seals Society
March of Dimes
Telephone Pioneers of America
Lions International
Kiwanis Clubs
Rotary Clubs
Sertoma Clubs
Optimist Clubs
Medicaid
Department of Health and Human Services
Commissions for deaf and hard of hearing people
Family service centers
United Way
Child health centers
Speech and hearing centers
Community centers and organizations for the deaf and hard of hearing
Church organizations
Hearing aid banks
Local charities

Another resource in the hunt for monetary help in purchasing hearing aids is HEAR NOW, a national program designed specifically to provide financial assistance to families and individuals with limited resources who need to purchase hearing-related devices. HEAR NOW maintains the National Hearing Aid Bank, which provides new and reconditioned hearing aids to deaf and hard of hearing people who can't afford to buy them at the retail price. If you'd like more information about the group and its programs, you can call (303) 695-4327 (TTY/ Voice) or visit the organization's website at http://www.leisureland.com/hearnow.

People who want to buy hearing aids and are looking for financial help can also check into hearing aid coverage from a private insurer. In the recent past, a number of state legislatures have introduced bills on that subject, and focus on the issue is growing steadily. In 2002 the state of Kentucky passed legislation that provided insurance coverage for hearing aids, joining Maryland, Oklahoma, and

Connecticut as the only states that provided some type of mandated insurance coverage for them. Insurance coverage for hearing aids will probably become more common as time goes on, and I encourage you to see what's available for you at the time you need it.

Feedback

One of the things you'll need to get used to when you start wearing hearing aids is the feedback they sometimes emit in the form of squeals or beeps. There's been considerable debate about whether or not a user of hearing aids should be told by someone else when his or her aids are making noise. In some quarters, it's considered impolite to mention the subject, while in others it's looked at as rude *not* to say something. Many users of hearing aids feel that if they can't hear the feedback their aid is emitting, they would prefer to be told about it in a polite way so they can spare those around them from any embarrassing or painful sounds. Trish Wilson, a late-deafened woman who wore hearing aids for years, and then got a cochlear implant, said that in her hearing aid days she wanted to be told "if I was whistling." When her hearing aids would start "singing" — which happened many times when she was in church — people nearby would begin to look around, wondering where the sound was coming from. When people began hunting for its source, Trish knew she should push her earmold in or turn down the volume on her aids to help stop the noise. She also pointed out that if people nearby knew her and were familiar with her hearing loss, and her aids started to beep, they'd usually smile and point to their ears. As Trish says "I sure did appreciate it!"

Not all feedback can be stopped by simply pushing in the earmold or turning down the volume on a hearing aid, of course. If neither work for you, take the unit to a hearing aid professional.

Tinnitus

Many late-deafened people have to deal with tinnitus or — as it's often called — "head noise." What about tinnitus and hearing aids? One late-deafened man says that his ongoing struggles with tinnitus are more successful with his hearing aids on since they "add some distracting noises." Another late-deafened individual, however, says that her hearing aids made her tinnitus markedly worse, especially if she entered a room where loud music was playing. Once exposed to music, she points out, "my ears would 'play' for me all day without respite." Like

Trish, she recently got a cochlear implant, and reports that it has eliminated much of the head noise associated with tinnitus, but says she still has to deal with it occasionally.

Questions and Answers

As I said at the beginning of this chapter, hearing aid use is a personal issue, and your experiences with your aids will undoubtedly be different from those of others who use them. Nevertheless, there are several questions and answers that can help virtually anyone who uses hearing aids or is thinking about getting them. Here are just a few.

Q. I've been told that the only really effective way to find the hearing aid that's best for me is to do a lot of hunting. Is that true?

A. Today's hearing aids offer an almost infinite range of options, and you can do a lot of exploring in order to find the aid that's best for you. Searching for the "right" one isn't really necessary (or practical) though. It's a lot more important to have the aid you buy properly adjusted to fit your specific needs.

◆   ◆   ◆

Q. Is there a way to obtain independent hearing aid research information instead of relying on the information hearing aid vendors provide?

A. Yes. Contact the Rehabilitation Engineering Research Center on Hearing Enhancement at Gallaudet University, 800 Florida Avenue NE, Washington DC 20002, an organization that conducts independent research on the subject.

◆   ◆   ◆

Q. The audiologists I've worked with tend to feature only the hearing aids of a few manufacturers. What should I do if I want to buy an aid that my audiologist doesn't offer or know much about?

A. Don't be too concerned about getting a specific brand. Nearly all people who need a hearing aid can be fit with a number of different kinds. Only individuals with an unusual hearing loss need to use a particular type.

◆   ◆   ◆

Q. My friend told me he had to try eight different kinds of hearing aids before he found the one that was right for him. Should I expect to go through something like that?

A. You could work that hard to find the right aid for you, but I'd suggest you spend the time finding the right person to fit your aids instead. As I said before, finding the aid that's right for you isn't all that difficult. It's more important to find an audiologist or hearing aid provider you feel comfortable with.

◆   ◆   ◆

Q. How about buying hearing aids without the help of a hearing specialist?

A. That would be a good way to save money, but your hearing is too important to take such a risk. You can't expect to replace the six years of studying it takes in order to become an audiologist with a little personal knowledge.

◆   ◆   ◆

Q. Hearing aids are so expensive, and many late-deafened people just can't afford them. Is anything being done about that?

A. Yes. At the time this is being written the International Federation of the Hard of Hearing is working on a solar powered hearing aid that's expected to cost about $55. Something like that would be affordable for virtually any potential hearing aid user.

◆   ◆   ◆

Q. What about telephone use with a hearing aid?

A. The chapter about telephone use for late-deafened individuals points out that all the major providers of telephone service claim to be accessible to hearing aid users. It's a good idea, though, to call your provider of telephone service and make sure that your needs will be met. It's also important to make sure that the design of your phone's headset is appropriate. The same is true of a Cochlear Implant (C.I.). If you decide to change to a C.I. after using a hearing aid, check to see if your telephone will work with one.

Looking For More Help?

If you love your hearing aids but want more help than they can provide, you may want to investigate the following option. Kathy Schlueter, the former president of the Association of Late-Deafened Adults, who talks about late-deafened grandparenting in the chapter about family and friends, reports that she uses a personal FM system — mentioned in the chapter about assistive devices — which can be attached to a hearing aid.

A hearing aid alone isn't enough for Kathy to hear as well as she'd like, but with the addition of the FM system her comprehension is far better than it would be without it. She especially likes that while attending a large meeting, she can ask an individual speaker to wear or hold her microphone and then pass it to each person who speaks.

Kathy's personal FM system is also extremely helpful when she's in an automobile. She loves that when she's riding in one others can wear her microphone and she can hear what's being said. Besides, as her kids told her a while ago, "thank God you don't have to turn your head as much as you used to so you could speechread us while driving."

Hearing Aid Care and Feeding

After you get one or two hearings aid, you'll want to get the most out of them. To do that, follow these simple guidelines:

- Educate your family and co-workers about how they can help you benefit from your aids as much as possible.

- Be careful not to let your aids get wet. Don't wear them in the shower, even under a shower cap.

- Keep them clean with rubbing alcohol, taking care not to get them too wet.

- Be sure to turn your aids off completely when they're not in use. You'll extend the life of both the aids and their batteries.

- When you go to the hairdresser, remove your hearing aids. Don't let them get wet, or wear them while you're sitting under the dryer.

- Remove your hearing aids when you go to bed, and, if needed to shut them off, remove the batteries as well.

- Keep a supply of extra batteries with you at all times. Murphy's Law definitely applies to hearing aids — the second you don't carry extra batteries, you can be sure the ones in your aid will run out.

- If you have a problem with your hearing aids, see your specialist as soon as possible. It's much simpler (and usually much cheaper) to deal with a problem with a hearing aid right away than later.

- Get the tubing in your BTE aids changed every six months or when it gets hard.

- Dogs and cats love the smell of ear wax, so don't leave your hearing aids where they can get at them. Canines and felines are also disturbed by high-pitched feedback from aids that haven't been completely turned off.

- If you have questions about almost any aspect of hearing aids, you can contact the Better Hearing Institute by telephone at (703) 684-3391 (V), in writing at Better Hearing Institute, 515 King Street, Suite 420, Alexandria, VA 22314, or by sending an e-mail to mail@betterhearing.org. If you have Internet access, you can check out the institute's web page at http://www.betterhearing.org/.

"I Can Hear Again!" — *Cochlear Implants*

When I was a child back in the Dark Ages (well, in the 1960s, actually), I learned that the best way to spark a lively discussion was to talk about sex, politics, or religion. After I went deaf in 1991, I learned that if you want to have an energetic discussion with a late-deafened person you should talk about cochlear implants. Why? Because many deafened people enjoyed minimal improvement with hearing aids and wanted an alternative. Then the cochlear implant (C.I.) came along, the alternative of their dreams had arrived. Most C.I. recipients — like grandparents when it comings to talking about their new grandkids — are more than happy to tell you about their implants.

Before we get too far into this chapter I want to issue a disclaim-er of sorts. I don't qualify for an implant because of my medical problems, so I consulted with two very knowledgeable C.I. users who answered my questions and read this chapter before it went to my publisher. Any oversights or factual errors in this chapter, however, are my responsibility, not theirs.

What's a C.I.?

If you already know what a C.I. is I promise I won't be offended if you skip this section. If you're in the mood for some exciting writing, though, you should keep reading this section (how's that for vanity?).

- A C.I. is a small and complex electronic instrument that can help a deaf or profoundly hard of hearing person hear sound.

- Although a C.I. is surgically installed in the brain, the insertion isn't very complicated. As someone who has had four surgeries on the brain tumor that caused my deafness, and has talked with a good number of C.I. users, I can attest that C.I. surgery is quite simple.

- A C.I. has four basic parts — (1) A microphone, which picks up sounds from the world around it; (2) A speech processor, which chooses and arranges the sounds picked up by the microphone; (3) A transmitter and receiver/stimulator, which receives signals from the speech processor and turns them into electric impulses; and (4) Electrodes, which gather the impulses in the receiver/stimulator and send them to the brain.

- A C.I. is very different from a hearing aid. A hearing aid amplifies all sounds so that people can hear them better, and a C.I. compensates for the parts of the inner ear that don't work. Technically speaking, a C.I. doesn't restore a user's natural hearing, but it does allow many users to understand speech and enjoy sounds of the environment.

- How many people have a C.I? On February 23, 2005 the National Institute on Deafness and Other Communication Disorders reported that 13,000 adults and nearly 10,000 children have a C.I. You can be sure that in the future significantly more kids and grown-ups will have them than do now.

A Brief Historical Overview

The first C.I. was developed during the 1950s by Andre Djourno, a French physiologist, and his assistant, Daniele Kayser, who were searching for a technique to stimulate nerves using a surgically implanted electrode. After successful experiments on animals, Djourno reasoned that a device that stimulated the auditory nerves might elevate human hearing, and began a collaboration with otolaryngologist Dr. Charles Eyries.

The initial C.I. patient was a man who had become deaf from an illness. On February 25, 1957, Eyries attached an electrode to the man's damaged vestibular nerve. Using a signal generator, the patient could hear limited sounds. Later, he was able to discern certain environmental sounds. The seeds of the modern C.I. had been sown.

Research on C.I.'s continued. Over the years, they went from single to multiple channels. By 1994 a speech-coding strategy and the Spectra 22 speech processor (with 22 channels) for the Nucleus system had been introduced by Cochlear Corporation. For some time, the Nucleus was considered the premier C.I. Then in 1995, the Food and Drug Administration approved the Clarion C.I., made by Advanced Bionics Corporation, which was very similar to the Nucleus except that its electrode array was curved rather than straight, which meant it could hug the wall of the cochlea better than the Nucleus. It also contained two "maps"

("maps" tells the C.I. how to work for each user) instead of one. Research has continued over the years, and C.I.'s have grown increasingly efficient.

Qualifications

Some people with residual hearing are afraid they won't be eligible for a C.I. because they're not "deaf enough." But there are at least two considerations used in determining who qualifies for a cochlear implant — first, a potential implant user must have a profound, bilateral sensorineural hearing loss and believe that he or she does not benefit significantly from hearing aids. In general, candidates for implantation must have tried hearing aids in the past and had little or no success with them. Second, he or she should generally be in good physical and mental health, although individuals with physical and psychological problems have received C.I.'s and enjoyed great success with them.

The Operation

In a C.I. surgery, general anesthesia is usually used. When the patient is "under," the surgeon or an assistant makes an incision in the skin and drills a hole in the patient's skull bone behind the ear. An electrode array is implanted in the cochlea and a receiver/stimulator is placed in the drilled-out area (a microphone, speech processor, and transmitting coil are worn externally and added later). The implant is secured with stitches, muscle, and tissue, after which the surgeon closes the incision and bandages the head. The surgery generally takes between three and six hours, during which time a surgical assistant monitors the facial nerve for any signs of facial paralysis. The hospital stay for a C.I. operation averages two days or less. But many C.I. patients receive an implant and are released the same day. Healing time is generally three to five weeks.

Expectations

C.I.'s have become considerably more sophisticated and successful in the last few years, and that trend will continue. Nevertheless, it's still important to have realistic expectations about what a C.I. can and can't do for you. For example, implants shouldn't be thought of as eyeglasses for the ears. While eyeglasses can often restore normal sight to the wearer, sounds heard with a C.I. may be difficult to understand. Remember, too, that C.I.'s don't solve a hearing problem — they bypass it by using stimulation of the electrodes implanted in the cochlea to reintroduce the signals usually carried to the brain by our auditory nerve fibers.

Results are generally determined by the extent of damage to the auditory nerve before implantation, which can't be determined prior to surgery. Nor do C.I.'s work the same for everyone — some people enjoy great benefits from theirs and others don't.

Some individuals opt for implants because they've tried hearing aids in the past, haven't gotten great results from them, and feel like they might as well try a C.I. Then they spend thousands of dollars on a device that might help them (and will definitely require lots more money for future upgrades and improvements). Although the success level of C.I.'s keeps rising, it's a good idea to ask yourself what you expect your C.I. to do for you, and how you'll react if that doesn't happen.

It's also a good idea to watch out for people (both deafened and hearing) who claim that everyone who's deaf or hard of hearing should get a C. I. They tend to sing the praises of C.I.'s and don't talk about the fact that C.I.'s simply aren't right for everyone with a hearing problem. People sometimes create unrealistic expectations for all C.I.'s because of their own experience with one, and it's a good idea to make up your own mind about getting an implant rather than depending on someone else who knows little about your particular needs, desires, or situation.

Related to that is the issue of family members and friends who want you to get a C.I. because they think that it will make you "hearing" again and you can have regular conversations with them again. While it's perfectly understandable for loved ones to want you to be like you always were, C.I.'s aren't some kind of magic pill that will restore your hearing. Sometimes they work well enough to allow you to participate in everyday conversation, and other times they don't. Only you can decide whether or not you should — and want to — get one.

Costs

How much should you expect to pay for a C.I? The cost can vary widely from hospital to hospital and year to year. For example, in 2000 one late-deafened woman paid $45,000 for hers, and said C.I. prices at the hospital where she got her implant ranged from $30,000 to $60,000 depending on what kind of equipment a recipient gets and how much "mapping" (programming after the operation) is required. Exact prices are not only a result of each hospital's differing fees, but are also determined by the amount of accessories a patient's audiologist orders with the main implant device.

Unless you're independently wealthy, you'll probably need help from your insurer to pay for your C.I. There's a trick, though — some insurers still consider C.I. surgery "experimental," and refuse to pay for it. Similarly, Medicare, a federal health insurance program for Americans over 65 and younger disabled people, usually pays only a portion of the cost of C.I. surgery.

A prominent doctor once pointed out that although cochlear implant surgery involves opening up the head, it isn't very complicated. In his words, the surgery is "not a terribly big deal." So the question for a lot of potential C.I. recipients is this — if the surgery isn't considered all that intricate, why is getting an implant so expensive? Several factors influence the final cost. Here are a few.

Support Services

Part of the high price of a cochlear implant results from the support services an implant user receives. To cite just one example: surgeons, C.I. patients, and audiologists can all call Cochlear Corporation and get a rapid reply to questions they have. The cost of this support influences the final price of a C.I.

Research and Development

Although the technology to manufacture cochlear implants has been available for many years, C.I. manufacturers have had to avoid the "breast implant" syndrome in which silicone breast implants occasionally leaked into the body and caused negative immune system reactions. Cochlear implant manufacturers need to ensure that the implanted device is made of durable material that will not deteriorate when it comes in contact with body fluids and chemicals. They also must ensure that the body will not reject the device and that the device won't be damaged in the wide range of human activities. As a result, cochlear implant makers spend a great deal of money on research and development.

Marketing

Food and Drug Administration regulations prohibit television advertisements for cochlear implants in the United States. Unlike many makers of medicine and medical equipment, implant manufacturers can't leave a sample of the device for doctors to dispense. As a result, they must advertise in appropriate media instead, which can cost a substantial amount.

Warranty Servicing

Replacing a speech processor under warranty can be expensive, and the cost of warranty servicing figures in the final price of an implant. The cost, like all C.I.-related support services, is borne by implant recipients.

Lack of Competition

The price of implants is also a product of the large market share the principal implant manufacturers have today. In the past, Cochlear Corporation enjoyed a virtual monopoly in the C.I. market, but the introduction of the Clarion C.I. by Advanced Bionics Corporation changed that considerably, although competition is still minimal. When the manufacture of high-quality cochlear implant systems becomes more commonplace, the price of C.I. implantation may come down.

Personal Experiences

That's enough technical talk. One of the best ways to figure out if a C.I. is right for you is to read the stories of some deafened people who have one. So below are the stories of several individuals who have implants.

Debra Charles

Debra suffered from a progressive hearing loss because the hairs in her cochlea were dying off. She was growing increasingly frustrated at her inability to find a well-paying job as a deaf person, so she received a cochlear implant in January of 1992, when the C.I. was still fairly young. The results were excellent. When asked if she would get one again, she says emphatically that she would get one even sooner than she did so she could avoid spending so many years of her life working in low-paying jobs that didn't challenge her.

Getting a C.I. also brought Debra some real personal satisfaction: "people are much more willing to communicate with me now," she points out.

When asked about her expectations for the implant, Debra said she hoped her C.I. would allow her to speechread better and maybe hear on the telephone a little. Did that happen? "Absolutely!" Debra said. She also has noticed a marked improvement in her speechreading skills because of her C.I., and now she can use the telephone in the usual way.

What does Debra like best about her C.I? "That I can hear on the phone again." The worst, she reports with a smile, is that sometimes the batteries in her

C.I. run out at the wrong time (is there a right one?). She's learned, though, to carry extras with her all the time.

Carolyn Piper

Carolyn decided to get a cochlear implant several years ago because she had reached the point where she could hear almost nothing with the strongest hearing aids. Even then, she put off getting a C.I. for "a couple years" until the C.I. center in her area had done the procedure on a few people first.

Having worked in a hospital for years before she got her C.I., Carolyn had a fair amount of skepticism in terms of expectations for any medical procedure. She feels this was fortunate in the case of her C. I., because her doctor tends to lead many of his patients to expect excellent results from an implant, and she was able to evaluate accurately the potential benefit of getting one.

Being fully aware of the mixed results of cochlear implants, Carolyn's goals for her C.I. weren't unrealistic — she was simply hoping to regain the ability to hear enough to function one-on-one and interpret environmental sounds again. These goals have largely been met, although in face-to-face situations she continues to have trouble understanding people if they don't speak slowly and modulate their speech.

Still, like Debra, Carolyn has no doubts that she would get a C.I. again if she had to choose. As she points out, "my verbal understanding is still very imperfect...but I have regained my confidence in approaching people one-on-one, which I had been losing while using bilateral hearing aids."

Carolyn also doesn't hesitate when asked what she likes best about her C.I. — knowing that her hearing is essentially stable now. "Even though I was profoundly deaf while wearing hearing aids," she recalls, "I could always detect an almost daily fading in my hearing ability. That's no longer happening."

On the flip side, Carolyn says the hardest thing about getting a C.I. was seeing so many family members and friends "hurt for me" when her results didn't meet the expectations they had. Many of Carolyn's friends felt that a C.I. would restore her previous level of hearing, and were disappointed when it didn't.

Bill Graham

Bill is a co-founder of the Association of Late-deafened Adults (ALDA) and the former executive director of Hearing Loss Link. He was deafened over a period of 20 years, and when growing up was told by his mother "not to make a mountain out of a molehill" with regard to his hearing difficulty.

For Bill, though, his hearing problem was more than a "molehill." After a journey of many years during which he alternately bluffed that he was hearing, learned sign language and socialized with Deaf and deaf people, and immersed himself in ALDA, he opted for a C.I. in 1995. Why? Because studies and personal observations have suggested that C.I. technology had greatly improved over the years. Bill also reports that the implant and moving from his hometown of Chicago to the Pacific Northwest has changed his life markedly; he seldom encounters sign language in social or professional situations now. In addition, Bill and his wife Karina now have two adopted hearing children, and he wants to be able to with them communicate as well as possible.

Bill characterizes his C.I. experience as a great success. He can now use the telephone fairly effectively, although he has never gotten into the habit of talking on it any more than sporadically. He can identify and enjoy simple (non-orchestral) music he knew as a youngster, but has trouble following unfamiliar music. He sometimes listens to audio books on tape when he's driving, walking, or jogging by himself, and credits a lot of his improvement with his C.I. to this practice.

Bill no longer uses sign language interpreters at work meetings, preferring to use his C.I. and assistive listening devices. His greatest appreciation of his C.I., however, is on the home front, where the device brings in loud and clear the "sing-song voices" of his two young children.

Bill reports that he'd definitely have C.I. surgery again. In fact, he says he's thinking of getting a C.I. for his other ear. As he reported recently, C.I. technology has improved steadily since he got his first C.I. in 1995, and evidence suggests that bilateral implants can reduce the problem of background noise, which he calls "my greatest bugaboo."

Bev Biderman

A deafened woman from Canada, Bev Biderman is a truly uncommon cochlear implant recipient. Her C.I. was "turned on" on July 8th of 1993, and she's had excellent results with it, but what's truly impressive is that she shared her implant story with the world by writing a book called <u>Wired for Sound — A Journey Into Hearing</u>. It not only details her very positive personal experiences with her C.I., but also addresses several other issues, including deafness in the family, the attitude of Deaf people toward C.I.'s, and the future of implants. Robert Shannon, the Ph.D. who directs the auditory implant research laboratory at the House Ear Institute has called Bev's book "a thoughtful and moving story" of the challenges that come from being deaf. C.I.'s may be medical devices, but

Biderman's book captures, as Shannon says, "the full personal human and social story of the impact of such devices on people who get them and on their families and friends." Larry Orloff, the editor of the magazine *Contact*, calls <u>Wired For Sound</u> "the most extensive compilation of resources relating to cochlear implants that I have seen," and Susan Goldberg, a professor of psychology and psychiatry at the University of Toronto, reports that the book's combination of personal experience and detailed information makes for "compelling reading." Goldberg reports she "didn't want to put it down." If you're thinking about getting a C.I. you want to check out "this very readable book."

Cheryl Heppner

The executive director of the Northern Virginia Resource Center for Deaf and Hard of Hearing Persons, Cheryl Heppner, received a cochlear implant in March of 2000. The former president of the Association of Late-Deafened Adults points out that her first experience with a C.I. was, as she puts it, "not one of the grand successes." The required surgery went fine, but she had a difficult recovery from it because of problems tolerating the required post-operative medications she had to take. She also noted that her "reprogrammings" — a regular requirement for C.I. users — didn't help her for long. Her brain adapted very quickly to any new "maps" in her processor, and they became ineffective. For instance, after being reprogrammed, there would be a week or two when her brain was adjusting to the new settings, and then the programs would lose their effectiveness. Sometimes it seemed like she was experiencing an overnight loss, but she suspects that there was a steady, gradual decline until she simply couldn't hear as many things as she did as when she was first reprogrammed.

Still, Cheryl is sure she would opt for a C.I. again if she had to choose. She can now monitor her own voice much better than she could in the past, and reports that the ability to do so has improved markedly since receiving her C.I. She is also enjoying music again, and says it's not nearly as painful to be stuck in traffic when you can listen to a C.D. She also points out that her brain continues to adapt to her C.I., and feels that she can now pick up more complexity in what she hears. Cheryl also reports that sometimes she can even understand people without looking at them when they talk in a quiet environment and she can do a little guessing. She says that "despite the frustration of the setbacks, I have had so much enjoyment and fun."

Lori Heir

Lori is the newest C.I. user profiled in this chapter — so new, in fact, that her C.I. was installed but not "hooked up" (i.e. turned on) when this chapter was written. So I can only share her hopes and expectations regarding her implant with you.

That's start wit a little history. Lori began losing her hearing in 1992 when she was almost 17. At first it was a mild loss. Then she woke up completely deaf one morning in May of 2003.

Lori's expectations for her C.I. are relatively low. She's hoping to be able to hear environmental sounds like horns and sirens for safety reasons. She would also like to hear speech and music, and have usual telephone conversations (not with a TTY), but is keeping her hopes in check. Lori feels that hearing sound again will be a pleasant surprise, but if the C.I. doesn't work, she will go on leading a very happy life as a deaf person.

Lori told me she thinks that her mother just wanted her daughter to come through the surgery without any complications. So she was very happy that happened. Mom isn't sad that Lori can't hear, and just accepts her daughter for who she is. Lori thinks Mom just doesn't understand why Lori is opting for a C.I., but it's very clear how much Lori's mom loves her daughter. A few months after Lori lost her hearing, her mother wrote the following poem, which expresses exactly how she felt about her daughter's post-deafness life.

A Desire to Admire
by
Jerilyn Heir

She awoke in the night
And came running to say,
"I can't hear my own voice!"
In tears and a cry, and hearing all gone,
Without any choice.

What could I do? What could I say,
To help my daughter believe it'd be ok?
When in my own heart,
I thought it was awful.
I stared into space, and held her so tight.

I prayed take my hearing in serious fright.
How would she do it? How could I help?

Not right away, but changes did come.
I watched her grow stronger
And fear deafness no longer.
She lives with desire —
there's nothing she can't do
and everything to admire.
in a world that became silent.

Her calling she heard.
That night when she woke up
And called out my name,
In fear and in pain,
And with terrible shame,
Of the loss that she suffered
And a future unknown,
It's all but a blur now
And hard to believe

We once only could grieve.
Now there's nothing to grieve,
But only things to enjoy,
And half the joy is watching
My daughter awake
To a world she's only
Just begun to embrace.

Is there a bottom line when it comes to cochlear implants? Nope. Do your "homework," talk with people who have a C.I., and then make a decision about getting one based on what you know and how you feel. If you run into someone — regardless how close to you — who thinks differently than you about your getting a C.I. consider the title of a play that was popular several years ago — *Whose Life Is It Anyway?*

FAMILY & FRIENDS

The chapter about the psychology of late-deafness talked about the challenges people face in their emotional lives after they lose their hearing. That's particularly true of interactions with family members and friends. When you go deaf, the easy communication with others that you've enjoyed for years becomes a thing of the past, and many people you're close to simply won't know how to treat you. As a result, they'll sometimes avoid you as much as possible.

Other individuals, fortunately, will have no problem meeting your particular communication needs. That seems to be especially true of younger people. For instance, many of my nieces and nephews see my use of a laptop computer or other electronic device as a principal means of communication with them as "cool." As a result, we have some great conversations. Unfortunately, lots of my relatives and friends — particularly those who've known me for a long time — have resisted the changes my deafness has caused, and have silently but very obviously turned away from me since I went deaf. You might encounter something similar, since people who've known you for a long time are often set in their ways and are resistant to changing what they believe.

Speaking of that, there's something to watch out for when it comes to deafness and your relatives and friends. Lots of the people you've known for a long time will want you to hear again after you go deaf, and will urge you to get strong hearing aids or a cochlear implant so they can communicate with you easily. I'm hardly in a position to tell you if either is right for you, and I'll leave that to you and your medical team. What I want to do instead is offer some simple strategies to help make your post-deafness relationships with family and friends as rewarding as possible.

Some People Just Won't "Get It" — and You Shouldn't Expect Them To

Before you start taking the steps needed to maintain good relationships with family members and friends after you go deaf it's important to realize that many of them just won't "get it" when it comes to deafness. That doesn't mean they're bad people — they simply don't see the connection between hearing and so much in life. You really shouldn't expect them to, either. After all, most family members and friends of late-deafened people have never been deaf themselves or known anyone who is, and they couldn't possibly fathom what it means to live without sound. Similarly, there are all sorts of things many late-deafened people — especially if they've been deaf for several years — don't really understand with regard to life with normal hearing, such as communicating easily with others, using the telephone in the usual way, appreciating the beauty and subtleties of the human voice, and on and on. That isn't good or bad — it just *is*. Both hearing and deaf people simply don't "get" certain things that are beyond their understanding, and it's a good idea to accept that fact rather than fighting against it. Besides, research has shown that hanging onto a grudge can increase our chronic stress levels. While the chapter on the psychology of late-deafness pointed out that stress is sort of an inevitable part of life for most deafened people, the chronic kind raises blood pressure, which may lead to premature arterial aging. Late-deafened people already have plenty to deal with because of their inability to hear, and they don't need to add extra stress to their lives by expecting hearing friends or family members to understand what it's like to live without sound.

It's also important to remember that when a friend or family member "loses it" on you after you go deaf it may not have anything to do with you or your inability to hear. You may simply be the recipient of the anger or frustration that the person feels about someone or something in his or her life, or the inability to communicate easily with you. While it can be difficult to deal with a blow-up by someone who's important to you, don't forget that the only person who really understands your needs, desires, and circumstances is you. Easily said, but hard to do, huh? Well, here are some tips to make it a little easier for you to maintain good relationships with family members and friends after you go deaf.

Beware of Personalization

For starters, be sure not to personalize others' reactions or outbursts. There's really no way of telling what went on in another person's recent past or how he or she is dealing with it. How they treat you at any given time may just be a product of that — and have nothing to do with you or your deafness.

Another important thing to do when someone blows up at you is to ask yourself a simple but important question: "How much power am I willing to surrender to others?" When we place a higher value on other individuals' actions and consider their reactions and attitudes more important than our own feelings, we belittle ourselves. There are plenty of things in the world that have the potential to make us feel small, but we don't have to give in to any of them. So keep your mind on the reality of the present and don't obsess about others' feelings. Other people's unhappiness or "disease" is their problem — don't make it yours.

Reach Out

One of the first steps you'll need to take with friends and family members after going deaf is to reach out to them. Many hearing people will feel uncertain about whether or not they should try to communicate with you after you go deaf, and even fewer — if they decide to stay in touch with you — will know how best to do so. So it's up to you to assure them that although your ears don't work anymore you're still perfectly capable of giving and receiving love and friendship.

Don't just tell them that, though. SHOW THEM! Remember that old saying about actions speaking louder than words? That's really applicable when your hearing decides to call it quits. As I pointed out above, most hearing people won't know how to communicate with you after you lose your hearing, and — as a result — may go silent on you. So you need to reach out and show them through your actions that you still care deeply about them. Send a card or letter, or set up a time to talk with them, whether on the telephone or in an on-line chat room. Do whatever it takes to assure others that communicating with them — although it poses some obstacles now — is important to you. That will make both you and them feel much more secure and will increase the opportunity for genuine interaction between you.

Get Used to Not Knowing Things

It's been more than a decade since I lost my hearing, and although there are some things I'm glad I don't have to listen to anymore (rap music and voice mail are at the top of the list!), I've also gotten used to the fact that there are certain things I'll simply never be told. Several times since going deaf I've been the recipient of the dreaded "it wasn't important" phrase when I said "what?," and more than once I simply wasn't told something in the first place because doing so would have required more effort than the speaker wanted to expend. That, unfortunately, seems to be especially common with friends and family members. Almost everyone feels they're busy, and taking the time to really communicate with a late-deafened person is generally out of the question for them. There doesn't seem to be any solution for that, so it makes sense for a late-deafened person to simply get used to not knowing certain things. I'm not suggesting that we settle for a lack of knowledge when it comes to important issues, such as doctor's instructions — a subject I talked about in the chapter on communication — but it's a good idea to accept the fact that family and friends often feel they simply don't have the time needed to tell you everything you want to know. Like hearing people often not understanding deafness, that doesn't mean they're "bad" people — just that communicating with you after you go deaf is often too time-consuming for them.

Although it can be frustrating not knowing something that goes on around you, there are also great benefits in it. Yes, there are things we need to know about, and at times like that it's important to be assertive and get the information that's important to us. But all the time? Nope! Do we really need to know about Aunt Bertha's new dishtowels, for example, or hear the latest gossip about a neighbor? I doubt it. We need to accept that there are some things we as deafened people will simply never know about our family members and friends. That doesn't mean that we're not a good friend to someone or an unimportant part of our family — just that we're different from other people. Part of being deaf is not being privy to everything that goes on in our world.

That's true for everyone, though. No one — whether hearing or deaf — can possibly know everything that happens in his or her world. We like to tell ourselves that the opposite is true, but the fact is that everyone has certain subjects they know little or nothing about. Why not simply accept that reality? That would surely bring us a lot of peace, and allow us to preserve our energy for things we can influence.

Listen Up

When you go deaf, it's important to listen closely to family and friends. No, this isn't a joke, or some kind of pitch for hearing aids or cochlear implants. It's about listening, not hearing. While late-deafened people can't do the latter anymore, they're definitely still capable of the former.

How are hearing and listening different? These definitions from Webster's New World Dictionary sum it up perfectly. "Hearing," the dictionary tells us, is a purely physical activity, "the act or process of perceiving sounds." To listen, by contrast, is the emotional activity of paying close attention. Quite a difference, huh? When it comes to your relationships with family members and friends, isn't listening much more important than hearing?

If you talk with members of a couple that's been together for years, and you ask them the secret of their relationship's longevity, one or both partners will almost always point to the outstanding communication between them. If you ask one partner to explain that further, he or she will usually talk about what a good listener the other partner is.

How does a late-deafened person improve his or her listening skills? Simple — by paying closer attention to what others are really saying, whether it's through spoken words, sign language, or written communication. Rather than simply being sure of what words the other person is using, focus on what he or she means. Instead of striving only to understand what's said, signed, or written, pay attention to the speaker's facial expression, posture, and body language as well. There may be quite a big difference between what's said and what's meant, and the latter is much more important.

Doing that in everyday life is important, of course, but it's particularly important in our relationships with family and friends. When you take your car in for an oil change, or are conversing with the person who's painting your house, focusing on factual information makes perfect sense. When you're talking with a friend or relative, though, you need to pay attention to the feelings behind the spoken, signed, or written words.

Being a good listener requires you to turn your focus away from yourself and toward the speaker. You also have to avoid the habit of finishing the other person's sentences in an effort to save time or prove you've understood him or her. That can be difficult, especially in our "hurry-up" society, where we're often too busy to make time for real interaction with others. The pay-off, though, is tremendous: do it, and many of the issues in your relationships with friends and family members will disappear.

Keep Good Company

In some cases late-deafened people know very few others, and as a result feel "beggars can't be choosers." I can definitely relate. Although many of the people I know will do whatever it takes to communicate effectively with me now that I can't hear, there were also some folks who were at a total loss when I went deaf. As a result, our friendship sort of disappeared along with my hearing. We're still nice to each other, but there's no question that my deafness has changed our relationship markedly.

You've probably experienced that too. After you went deaf, some of your family members and long-time friends probably "freaked out," and now avoid you as much as possible. Unfortunately, that's quite common. There doesn't seem to be a lot you can do about that. Some people simply don't realize that things have to change if they want to maintain contact with you after you lose your hearing. But don't despair. Just do your best to keep good company. Hang onto the long-time friends who are willing to deal with your deafness, and welcome new friendships with people who see that your inability to hear doesn't have to be an obstacle to connecting with you in a meaningful way.

Maintaining friendships isn't just an emotional issue either. A study I read about recently found that people who enjoyed a high level of social well-being because of supportive friends and neighbors had a considerably lower level of vascular endothelial growth factor in their blood. While there's some question of what this compound does, it's generally thought to contribute to the growth and proliferation of cancer cells. So keeping it low may help you stay healthy.

Embrace Change

While it's important to reach out and let people know that your going deaf doesn't have to interfere with your relationships with them, you also shouldn't be afraid to move beyond what you're used to. The following piece is a great reminder of how important it is to welcome change.

Before I share it with you, I want to provide a little background. A few years after I lost my hearing, I discovered an on-line service called "Your Life Support System" (YLSS). Run by minister Steve Goodier (who writes all the material that appears on it), YLSS offers one-minute readings that warm the readers' hearts, and makes them think and feel (and laugh regularly too!). If you'd like to subscribe or learn more about the service, visit the Internet address http://www.lifesupportsystem.com.

A while ago, YLSS ran a piece about change, which struck me as particularly appropriate for late-deafened individuals. So I contacted Steve and got his permission to share it with you.

◆   ◆   ◆

EVERYTHING CAN BE DIFFERENT
by
Steve Goodier

Arizona Highways magazine once reported a funny sign spotted at the Road Runner Market in Quartzsite, Arizona. A sign on the counter read:

"Your patience is appreciated.
New electronic cash register.
Same old ladies."

Apparently, the business machines were changing faster than the clerks! Which isn't to say that people can't change. They can. In fact, our greatest hope is birthed from knowing that we CAN change. We don't have to remain the same. Things can be different than they are.

Nobody else can change your life. It is something only YOU can do. New and beautiful things await those who believe that things can be different. I've known relationships to improve dramatically once the couple learned this simple axiom: "You can't change your partner; but your partner can change." We change because we want to and because we believe we can. There is great hope in that.

The unhappiest people change the least. They are not convinced they can start over! They often believe that they cannot truly be different and must continue leading unhappy lives forever. They should learn from snakes....

Snakes know about shedding the past and putting on something new. Old ways, old habits, old ideas, and old attitudes don't fit forever. Once outgrown, we can shed them and grow into a new skin. (Ever thought you'd be learning a life lesson from a snake?)

Everything will be different when you're different. It begins with two indispensable ingredients — desire and belief. Those who WANT to shed the old skin and who BELIEVE they can, will make needed changes. And they will be happy.

◆   ◆   ◆

Late-deafness is all about change. Why not embrace it and grow rather than fighting against it and stop moving forward?

Parenting After Going Deaf

Parenting after a hearing loss is a big challenge. Since my wonderful wife and I decided not to have kids (which I discuss in more detail below), I talked with a few late-deafened parents and asked them to share their thoughts about the subject of post-deafness parenting with me. Here are just a few of their observations and suggestions.

* *Michele Bornert* is the deafened mother of three young children. Two of them were born before she became deaf. One of the two was only six months old when Michele suddenly lost her hearing during her pregnancy for her third child.

Communication is the biggest challenge for Michele as a mother. Her children are too young to sign, and sometimes she feels cut off from her own kids because she can't communicate easily with them. Michele regularly struggles with feelings of inferiority brought on by her deafness, especially when she goes to some gathering or function and all of the parents are chatting and getting to know each other while she's left alone. Sometimes she feels like she's not a good mother because she's different.

Michele sees some big benefits in being a deafened parent, though. At the top of her list are those car rides with her family. When you're a deaf parent you don't have to listen to your kids whining or yelling. It's really funny for her to look over at her husband while he's driving with the kids in the car and find him beet-red and clutching the steering wheel with both hands so tightly that his knuckles are white. "What's wrong?" Michele will ask him as she calmly flips through a magazine. He just looks over at her like he could kill someone at any moment (sometimes she doesn't know who he wants to kill more — the kids for screaming or her for being oblivious to the racket!).

Her children are still very young, so Michelle hasn't had to skip any of their concerts, games, and so on because she's deaf. She's had occasions, however, where they have had programs or Parent's Day at her kids' schools and the children wanted her to go, but she felt uneasy about doing so. At her son's Parent's Day, which happens every month, the school is happy to hire a professional interpreter. Her daughter's school, however, doesn't have the money to pay someone to interpret for Michele, and its leaders don't know of any parent who signs and would be willing to volunteer. Michele would like to go to all of her kids' special occasions — if nothing else, to give her support — but she knows that she can only handle so much of not understanding what's said. As she says, though, "if they have an interpreter, I'm there!"

Since becoming deaf, Michele's stopped taking her kids to the doctor and has turned the job over to her husband. She knows that really irritates him at times, but unless she can get an interpreter she'd feel unintelligent and like a burden.

Is there a specific strategy Michele follows to help her take an active role in her kids' lives? Sort of. She often tries to communicate with her children's teachers by sending them notes in the kids' backpacks. The teachers almost always reply with a note of their own. She also relies heavily on her husband to get essential information about her children's education.

Michele's decision to get a cochlear implant, which she received soon after her third child was born, was made hastily and didn't include much preliminary testing. When the implant was turned on it didn't help her at all. So she doesn't wear hers now.

* *Mary Clark* has been very active in the Association of Late-Deafened Adults (ALDA) for more than a decade, serving as its president twice. She and her husband Jeff have three daughters age 18, 15, and 9, all hearing. The 18-year-old and the 15-year-old were still very young when Mary lost her hearing, and the nine-year-old was born after her mom became deaf.

What's the biggest challenge Mary faces in being a late-deafened parent? To get her kids to communicate with her in a way she can understand. She didn't sign well immediately after she became deaf, and her kids were too young to fingerspell or write for her. She felt it was important for her to think positively about becoming deaf, though, so the girls wouldn't look at it as a depressing, negative thing.

Each of Mary's children has a different method of communicating with her, just as they have different personalities: they sign, fingerspell, or write. It's been a challenging journey for Mary to work with each of her kids in order to get the communication she needs and wants.

What's the biggest benefit of being a deafened parent? Not having to hear the noises she can live without — the radio, the whining, or the fighting in the car. Jeff often says he wishes he were deaf when he comes home from work and everyone is talking at the same time.

Has Mary stopped attending some of her kids' concerts, plays, sporting events, and so on because of her deafness? Yes and no. She does try to go to most of them or split them with her husband. The decision has nothing to do with her deafness, though. She simply doesn't attend things she's not interested in. She loves attending her kids' concerts and school plays, however, even if she can't hear anything, and her kids always ask their teachers for the scripts of their plays so Mom can follow along. Her children's events are very bittersweet for Mary, though: as much as she enjoys seeing her kids displaying their talent, she often sits in the audience and cries because she's so proud of her children but can't hear their sweet voices.

Mary and Jeff have also created some rules that have helped her be a better mother. One of them is that their kids must come to her to ask to do something, or to let her know their schedules. They used to go to their hearing father because that was easier for them. Mary often didn't know what was going on with her children, though, so now they must communicate with Mom first, who's in charge of the family calendar. The family also signs at dinner and when Mary is in the room. As Mary reports, "that doesn't always work, but we try." Another rule is that the captioning on the television set can never be turned off. They do occasionally bend that rule when the Chicago Bears play, though, because you can't always see the score if the captions are on. The family also has ALDA-Chicago parties at its house quite often, and Mary gives the girls various duties, such as serving soda, taking coats upstairs, and so on. This helps involve them in Mary's life and gives them opportunities to meet others who are deaf like their mom.

Mary doesn't think a cochlear implant would make her a better parent. It would be nice for her to be able to hear her children's voices, but she doesn't think that's necessary to be a good mom. She's learned to listen in different ways than hearing parents, and feels that as a mother she's very tuned in to her kids' body language and facial expressions. She's also certain to make "one-on-one" time for each child and do things they (and perhaps not she) are interested in. In addition — and very important to her — Mary always makes sure the kids know how much she loves them.

What's the first parental thing Mary would do if she could hear again? Have a party! She'd invite her kids' friends and the friends' parents over, and get to know them freely and without communication limitations.

* *Bill Graham*, the co-founder of ALDA, offers a special perspective on the issue of late-deafened parenting. He and his hearing wife Karina have adopted a boy and a girl with normal hearing who are six and four, respectively, as of this writing. Bill has a cochlear implant which allows him to communicate with his kids through spoken language, although there are moments when the kids are talking to an adult or other children and Bill can't understand what's being said. Communication problems also arise when the family's alone because the kids often choose to talk with their hearing mom rather than their late-deafened dad.

Another challenge for Bill is attending parental events such as conferences at school or birthday parties — the latter of which are typically noisy events —

because they make it difficult for him to communicate easily with others. At no other times does he feel so deaf.

Does Bill refuse to attend some of his kids' concerts, plays, sporting events, etc., because of his deafness? Not yet, although he often wants to skip them because of what he calls the "other-parents factor" (i.e. his inability to communicate with them). That can detract from the pleasure he gets from seeing his children in action.

His cochlear implant has pushed Bill into a different kind of limbo than other deafened parents, because at times he functions quite well with it, while in other situations he doesn't. Whereas in the past he might have planned strategies to help him deal with the problems his deafness caused (requesting real-time captioning, for example), he doesn't do that anymore.

Was Bill's decision to get a cochlear implant related at all to his desire to be a better parent? Partly, although he wanted to be able to hear in all sorts of situations, not just parenting.

What's the first parental thing Bill would do if he could hear normally again? Pick up his kids and the kids' friends and take them all to a baseball game.

The Flip Side — A Hearing Child with a Late-Deafened Parent

What's it like to be on the other side of the coin? Andoni Karavitis' mother Lynn started losing her hearing in 1997 when he was nine, and she's now almost totally deaf. Although Andoni is sad that his mom can't hear anymore, he told me that "life is not much different from when she could hear." Andoni feels some frustration because his mom went deaf, of course, but that's far outweighed by the comfort he feels because his mother is part of his life. As he puts it "It's not like I lost her because she lost her hearing." They both learned sign language after she went deaf, which allowed them to maintain communication with each other, and now they talk about all sorts of things, many of which have absolutely nothing to do with hearing.

It's not always easy for Andoni to have a late-deafened mom, of course, particularly if he needs to tell her something important. He also has some very real concerns about his deaf mom, such as her being alone in public. As he says, though, "My mom is still my mom, and nothing less. That will never change, hearing or not."

"Adopt" a Child Through the Mail

If real post-deafness parenting isn't possible or appropriate for you, you might want to consider an option that I've found particularly enjoyable: "adopting" a child through the mail. Sound kind of strange? Let me explain.

I was diagnosed with a brain tumor in April of 1987 at the "ripe old age" of 26, and while the ensuing surgery went very well my doctor told me afterwards that I would eventually go deaf because of the tumor. So I knew the inability to hear was coming. As a result, when I went deaf four and a half years later I was sad but not surprised.

Soon after that first operation (I've since had three more) I met Mary, and in just a few months I knew I wanted to spend my life with her. So I proposed, and she actually accepted (see, miracles do happen!). I also told Mary when I proposed that I didn't think we should have kids because of my tumor. Although neither of us liked that, it ended up being a wise decision, because about three years after she and I tied the knot the tumor took away not only my hearing but much of my balance and coordination, and left me with a truly horrid voice. So I wouldn't have made a very good dad.

That didn't mean Mary and I couldn't be parents of a sort, though. A few years ago, Mary and I adopted a child through the mail. Well, technically, we didn't adopt him. We sponsor him. What we do is send the non-profit agency Children, Incorporated a check every few months and they use it to buy the boy — an American Indian youngster who lives in Arizona — "frills" like food, clothes, and school supplies.

My deafness has been no obstacle to developing a relationship with our "adoptee," since the majority of our interaction with him happens via the mail. Many sponsors eventually meet the children they sponsor, and in September of 2001 Mary and I did exactly that. I can't think of many more treasured memories. If you'd like to find out more about the process of sponsoring a specific child through Children, Inc., you can write to the organization at P.O. Box 5831, 1000 Westover Rd, Richmond, VA 23220-0381, call 800-538-5381 (toll-free, voice) or (804) 359-4562 (voice), visit the Children Incorporated website at http://www.children-inc.org/main. html, or send a fax to (804) 353-4562.

Late-Deafened Grandparenting

Another important issue a number of late-deafened people face is that of being the best possible grandparent after going deaf. While not being able to hear can make grandparenting challenging, there are also some very simple steps you can take to be a big hit with your grandkids.

Kathy Schleuter, who served as the president of ALDA in 1999, is the grandmother of five, ranging in age from her grandson Brady, who's nine as of this writing, to her granddaughter Olivia, who arrived in 2002. Kathy was deaf when all of her grandchildren were born, so none of them had to adjust to a grandmother who went deaf after they'd gotten to know her. While it's frustrating for Kathy to watch her grandchildren try to tell her what their needs are or ask her a question, and not be able to do it effectively, she's also grateful for all the things they do together that don't have anything to do with hearing — coloring, baking, and working on puzzles, for instance. Sometimes she and Brady will type stories on the computer, search for clipart to use with the story, print the pages out, and then put them together in book form.

When I asked Kathy what specific recommendations she'd give to a late-deafened person who wanted to be as good a grandparent as possible, her answer was very clear: "love your grandkids unconditionally, just like we're asking them to love us and accept our hearing loss." For her, that means taking the extra time needed to be with them; reading, coloring, and playing games, and watching their activities. As Kathy says "we as late-deafened people may not hear everything that is going on during their activities, but to see grandma or grandpa in the crowd watching is letting the grandkids know we love them and want to be part of their lives."

She also makes another important point. As everyone knows, life is hectic and stressful at times for both adults and kids. As a grandparent you can be the one to take some pressure off a kid or bring more joy to him or her. Maybe you know sign language, maybe not, maybe you can speechread or not, but why not develop your own communication system with the youngsters? Kathy, for instance, doesn't ask for a full sentence in sign from her grandkids. As long as they can give her clues as to what they need, she can understand them well enough to be the kind of grandma every kid wishes he or she had. You can too.

ROMANCING THE STONE
(DEAF)

Think post-deafness love is a fantasy? Well, it's not. A hearing loss presents some significant challenges for couples in love or individuals seeking amour, but facing and overcoming them can yield real joy too. So in this chapter I want to talk about the issue of romance, love, and marriage after a hearing loss, and offer some tips to make your own post-deafness romantic experiences as rewarding as possible. Although my wife and I share a deep love for each other, I'm hardly an expert on the subject of love, and as with everything else in this book, I encourage you to look at what you read in the following pages through your own eyes and decide how to apply it to your life.

The Hearing-Deaf Divorce Myth

Let me start by debunking a particularly nasty fiction that's been around for years. It's been said that 90% of deaf-hearing unions (my wife and I jokingly call them "mixed marriages") end in divorce. That's not true. Here's how that fiction got started: years ago, an individual who was considered an authority on the subject of deafness was asked what he thought the divorce rate was in marriages where one partner is hearing and the other's deaf. After a few seconds, he guessed that it was about ninety percent. It was simple conjecture, but somehow it was taken as a fact. Then it stuck around. The reality, though, is that the failure rate of marriages in which one partner is deaf and the other is hearing is much lower than that guess. So if you or your beloved goes deaf, don't assume that your union is headed for the trash heap. What happens to one half of a couple is much less important than how both members react to it.

Don't Expect a Quick Fix

Many significant others of late-deafened people hope that hearing aids or a cochlear implant will take care of all of the problems that arise when their partner goes deaf. They won't, and it's unrealistic to expect them to. As the hearing husband of a late-deafened woman said a few years after her loss: "We realize now that hearing aids and cochlear implants aren't magic. They don't solve all your problems. Nothing does."

That includes sign language, speechreading, and cued speech. They can all be helpful, but there are no "miracle drugs" that will make a hearing loss — or the changes it brings — go away, or lead to an easy life. It's far wiser for the couple to accept the reality of a partner's loss, make whatever adjustments needed to maximize communication, and then get on with life.

Expecting a quick fix for a hearing problem also suggests a lack of appreciation for the late-deafened partner's other abilities. Significant others of late-deafened individuals might be tempted to focus on the fact that their partners can't hear anymore, but wouldn't it make more sense to think about what brought the two of them together in the first place? A few years ago I had a t-shirt made that said "it's about ability, not disability," which was a comment on both my acquired deafness and the physical deficits my brain tumor left me with. I realize now that's also an important philosophy for romantic success when half of a couple goes deaf. It's what a deafened partner can still do rather than what he or she can't do after going deaf that really matters.

"Hear" What Your Partner is Saying

In the chapter about post-deafness relationships with family members and friends I talked about the difference between hearing and listening, and the need to do the latter rather than simply hearing what others say.

That's particularly true when it comes to romantic relationships in which one of the partners goes deaf. As I pointed out in that chapter, people in long-term relationships usually mention how good a listener their partner is, and there's no reason a late-deafened person can't be one too. Take time to strengthen your listening skills, and you'll be amazed at how much that improves your romantic relationships.

What's the best way for a late-deafened person to become a better listener? Practice, more practice, and still more practice. Instead of worrying about the fact that you can't hear, focus on what the speaker means. Take into account the speaker's facial expression and body language when he or she's speaking. Do that regularly, and in time you'll become a really top-notch listener, even if your hearing is non-existent.

You Don't Always Have to Say Something

The flip side of listening to what your partner says is particularly good news for late-deafened people — that individuals in romantic relationships don't always have to say something to one another. Sometimes simply sitting together in total silence is the most romantic thing two people can do.

Couples in which one partner is late-deafened and the other is hearing may spend a lot of time together in silence just because of the difficulty of communication between them. In those situations, silence is usually an unwanted and inevitable response to an unpleasant reality. What I'd like to suggest, however, is making silence a conscious and positive choice that gives you and your significant other an opportunity to spend some very valuable time together.

Here's how it works, although you naturally can adapt the following to fit your particular interests.

- Sit next to each other in a comfortable position.
- Hold hands if you want, although that's certainly not required.
- Close your eyes and clear your mind as fully as possible.
- Breathe deeply, slowly, and peacefully. Don't worry about accomplishing anything. Just sit still and enjoy the moment.

How long and how often you do it is up to you. Although the process is quite simple, you'll be amazed at how profoundly and positively it affects your relationship and helps provide a sense of calm and strength that's particularly helpful when we butt against the craziness that everyday life often throws at us. It's a good idea to do it in the morning, perhaps after you've eaten breakfast or gotten your caffeine "fix," and before you head out the door.

What does such a simple activity do for a relationship? Lots! Most important, it allows the participants to share a powerful connection with one another. When couples spend time together simply breathing calmly, their defenses tend to disappear, and consequently they're more willing to open their hearts to one another. When the participants open their eyes after sharing such an experience, they generally feel considerably more loving towards the world. Best of all, their sense of love for — and connection with — their partner is strengthened.

Excessive Protectiveness

Several late-deafened spouses or significant others of hearing people have remarked that their hearing mates often try to protect them from the challenges of living in a silent world. While the desire to do so is admirable, it seems much healthier — for both the relationship and the late-deafened partner — to allow a deafened spouse or significant other to take responsibility for his or her own life. That doesn't mean that people in couples can't do positive things for one another, or take steps to protect a partner, of course, but it's a good idea to establish some ground-rules regarding what's acceptable. As one late-deafened spouse married to a hearing person put it a while ago "Education and awareness are key…. If both people are willing to communicate and say something like 'You're overstepping your boundaries,' it works."

Don't Expect Your Significant Other to Be Your Full-time Interpreter

Speaking of boundaries…My wife Marvelous Mary, who's both hearing and a certified interpreter for the deaf (so she's a much better signer than me), often translates what people say into sign language when we're both talking with them. That way I can follow the conversation much easier than if she didn't (my speechreading skills are almost non-existent). While I greatly appreciate that, I also realize that it's both unfair and unrealistic of me to expect her to do it all the time. She often wants to remain part of the conversation she's interpreting for me, and she really can't do that when she's signing what someone else in it says. Besides, she often spends much of her workday signing to others, and when she's away from her job she deserves a break from that. Most important, she also has a life of her own — and she can't enjoy it fully if I try to make her my full-time personal interpreter.

Don't Speak for Him or Her

Connected to the idea of not making a loved one your full-time interpreter is this — not speaking for him or her, or allowing him or her to do it for you. It's tempting for the significant others of late-deafened people to do so, because it often allows for easier (and faster) communication. Late-deafened partners of hearing people frequently speak for them too, because the "deafie" wants to a) prove that he or she has understood what's been said, and b) hang onto some kind of control in the relationship despite the inability to hear.

Those desires are certainly understandable, although I strongly recommend that you abandon the idea of speaking for someone else. There are a couple reasons for that.

The most obvious one is that people — both hearing and late-deafened — usually hate being spoken for. Partners who have endured that often say things like "I hate it when he speaks for me" or "It drives me crazy when she puts words in my mouth." What a great way to damage a relationship!

More than making a partner angry, speaking for him or her is a not-so-subtle sign of disrespect. Regardless of the speaker's intentions in doing so, speaking for a partner sends a message that the hearing half of the couple doesn't think the deafened person is capable of speaking for him or herself. It also implies that the speaker knows the late-deafened person better than he or she does. Can you imagine anything more unrealistic or irritating?

Speaking for someone else, particularly a person who's deaf, might make communication a little faster and easier, which is important to many people in today's world. It's also, however, extremely irritating to the person who's spoken for. The speed and ease it may create is nice, but such an action will almost always end up having a very negative effect on the relationship. You sure don't want that.

Don't Finish His or Her Sentences

Closely related to the idea of not speaking for someone you care about is one that I talked about in post-deafness relationships with family and friends — that of not finishing his or her sentences. Although doing so is common among both deaf and hearing people who have been married or in a relationship for a long time, resisting the temptation to do so will have a major — and very positive — impact on the quality of your interactions with the people you love.

Finishing other people's sentences is pretty common among late-deafened people, because we often think it accomplishes two things:

1) It proves that we've understood what's being talked about, and 2) It saves valuable time. As I said before, it takes much longer to do certain things when you can't hear, and many people regularly try to save a few seconds or minutes wherever they can. Interrupting someone and finishing other's sentences is simply one means of accomplishing that.

Although both reasons for finishing other people's sentences or interrupting them may appear to be logical, I strongly urge you to avoid both. Your partner will feel much more appreciated if you don't interrupt him or her, and that will certainly improve the quality of your relationship. It will also afford you a certain amount of inner peace because you won't have to be inside your partner's head trying to figure out what he or she is going to say.

Fortunately, retraining yourself not to finish others' sentences or interrupt them is easy. It's just a habit that needs to be developed. The next time you start to interrupt him or her, simply say to yourself (very gently, of course) something like "There I go again." Not only will that stop you from doing it now, but will also diminish your desire to do so in the future. You can also remind yourself before a conversation begins that you'll be patient and let others finish saying things. The people you communicate with — not only significant others, but friends and family as well — will feel closer to, and more comfortable with, you because they won't have to rush in order to avoid being interrupted. As a result, they'll be much more likely to share their feelings and thoughts with you. You can just imagine the positive effect that will have on both your everyday life and your romantic relationships.

Embrace Change

The chapter about friends and family talked about the need to accept change rather than fight against it. That's true when it comes to romance too. Having a spouse or significant other go deaf is obviously a big change, and many of us who lose our hearing hope (and sometimes expect) that our spouses or significant others will accept the new person who emerges. Sometimes that happens. In other cases, unfortunately, it doesn't. We've probably all heard stories about a spouse or significant other making a break for it when the person she or he was sharing life with went deaf. In fact, a while ago a good friend told me how his wife left him after he started developing a serious hearing loss, although it's easy to see that he's a very supportive and caring person, and probably treated his wife like a queen both before and after he started going deaf. Unfortunately, there doesn't seem to be a lot you can do about something like that. It appears to be an occasional and regrettable part of a relationship in which one partner goes deaf.

Fortunately, there are lots of heart-warming stories about spouses and significant others who stay with partners when the latter lose some or all of their hearing. I know they're not myths, because that's exactly what happened to me. My going deaf meant my wife and I had to change many of the ways we communicated with one another, but it also reminded us that the day would come when one of us would leave the earth, and that we should enjoy our time together while we could, regardless of the fact that one of us couldn't hear anymore. Besides, we were hopelessly in love with each other (and still are) and weren't going to let my inability to hear stand in the way of that.

Our Hearing Partners Change Too

In addition to being aware of the changes people undergo after losing their hearing, we need to remember something very important: that the partner of a newly-deafened individual also changes. Granted, most changes in life aren't as dramatic or drastic as going deaf, but that doesn't mean they're not important to the person who experiences them. Late-deafened people need to accept that everyone changes, and that the shifts they undergo can cause major alterations in a hearing partner's life too. While we often expect or hope that others will embrace our changes when we go deaf, we also need to make a genuine effort to accept theirs. Just think how much more pleasurable our romantic relationships would be if our partner felt free to change and knew that he or she would be loved and supported all the time, regardless of what those shifts were. What a wonderful recipe for long-term happiness!

Forget Traditional Gender Roles

When I was growing up in the 60's and 70's, there was sort of an unwritten law that said husbands were supposed to go to work and be the family's primary source of income, while wives stayed home, cooked, cleaned, and took care of the house's daily maintenance. If a couple decided to have children, the mother was expected to be responsible for most of the kids' up-bringing and day-to-day care. Some married women worked (usually part-time) but they were expected to be in charge of domestic matters while their husbands worked full-time in "real" jobs and focused on things like their careers.

That set of assumptions has changed markedly in the recent past, although some individuals still adhere to it. It sure doesn't apply to couples in which one partner goes deaf though, and I hope you'll abandon the notion.

For the first few years of our marriage, my wife and I followed that philosophy. She worked part-time as a freelance interpreter for the deaf, and I worked full-time (and then some!) as a college professor and department chairman. Although it was never stated outright, there was kind of an unspoken assumption that my career was more important than hers. A couple years after we tied the knot, in fact, we moved hundreds of miles from our friends and families in Connecticut so I could take a position chairing the theater department at a college in Georgia. Things changed dramatically after I went deaf in December of 1990, though. In addition to going deaf, the brain tumor that caused me to lose my hearing also gave me the "gifts" of terrible balance, coordination, and speech. So despite my desire to keep working after I wet deaf, there was simply no way I could.

We still needed a decent income, though, because the disability insurance and Social Security payments I got after my losses weren't nearly enough to support two people. Fortunately, Mary was soon offered a position as a sign language interpreter for a Deaf man in the U.S. Department of Education. So we packed up and moved north. In a few years, she became the manager of the department's interpreters, and later became a program specialist there. Today, although I still get social security benefits and disability insurance payments, Ms. Marvelous is our principal wage earner. I'm really just a "house-husband."

Although many late-deafened people continue to work after losing their hearing, largely because of the Americans With Disabilities Act, mine and Mary's experience is fairly common. Sometimes a spouse has to become the primary wage-earner in the family when his or her mate goes deaf. So accept the fact that traditional gender roles don't apply when one spouse enters the world of silence. Going deaf involves a lot more than a simple physical change, and it's important to embrace that reality.

Don't Make Him or Her Your "Punching Bag"

Imagine this — your boss growls something that you don't understand, the clerk at the grocery store says something you can't figure out (and repeats it three times without writing it down after you explain you're deaf), or your kids submit your sanity to a serious test. You're steaming. Then you meet your spouse or significant other. Take a wild guess who you choose to "lose it" on.

Venting generally isn't a big problem, and we all do it at times. It's just a part of life. I firmly believe, however, that doing so frequently with a spouse or significant other isn't a good idea.

Although it usually makes the person who does it feel a little better, repeated "venting" can have a very negative effect on the recipient and, hence, the relationship. For instance, your mate may be in a pretty decent mood before your explosion, but talking with you for a few minutes will change that drastically. While spouses and significant others can usually see very readily when a partner is in a bad mood, and can — hopefully — avoid developing one themselves, a certain amount of transference is inevitable. After listening to you rant for a few minutes, he or she will pick up some of the anger and frustration you feel. Do you really want to do that to someone you care about?

It's also unrealistic to expect the person who listens to your rant to offer much in the way of helpful suggestions. If you're upset about something that happened at work, for example, chances are slim that he or she will really understand how you feel. If your rant is related to your hearing loss, and he or she has never experienced one, there's simply no way your significant other can understand how you feel, and it's unrealistic of you to expect otherwise.

Instead of blowing up, you might want to try a technique that's expressed very well in a story I read a while ago:

◆   ◆   ◆

THE TROUBLE TREE

I decided to restore my house, so I hired a handyman to take care of some of the work. If his first day of work was any indication of what was to come, I wouldn't have blamed him at all if he had told me there was no way on God's green earth that he'd stay on the job.

For starters, a flat tire made him arrive an hour late. When he got to my place his electric saw didn't want to work. Then when lunchtime rolled around he found he'd forgotten his mid-day food at home.

The "fun" wasn't over though — at the end of the day his pickup decided it didn't want to start. So I drove him home. While I did that he sat in stony silence, and the look on his face suggested he wanted to strangle someone.

We arrived at his place, and he invited me in to meet his family. As we walked toward the front door, he stopped for a few seconds at a small tree in front of the house, touching its trunk with both hands.

We got to the front door, and the man proceeded to open it. When he did that, he underwent an amazing transformation. He suddenly had a big smile on his face, hugged his two small children, and gave his wife a warm kiss. Then he happily introduced me to the three of them.

After a little small talk, he walked me to my car. We passed the tree he'd stopped at before, and my curiosity got the best of me. So I asked him about what I had seen him do earlier. "Oh, that's my trouble tree," he replied. "There are times when I have a terrible day, and I feel awful, but I don't have to inflict that on my wife and children. So I just hang my troubles up on that tree when I come home. Then in the morning I pick them up again. The odd thing, though," he said with a smile, "is that when I come out in the morning to pick 'em up again, there aren't nearly as many as I remember hanging there the night before."

◆　　　◆　　　◆

There are lots of challenges in a life without hearing, and sometimes they leave us feeling depressed, angry, or both. That's just part of life, though. As the story above points out, we don't need to inflict our unhappiness or irritation on others, especially those we love. Why not develop a "trouble tree" of your own that lets you get rid of your frustrations instead of allowing them to affect your relationships?

Laugh at Yourself

It's no secret that I love to laugh. I'm also a big believer in the emotional and physical benefits of laughter. In fact, before I wrote this book I put together a collection of humor entitled He Who Laughs Lasts, which started with a foreword by the well-known M.D. Bernie Siegel and an introduction about the physical and emotional values of humor. I make a concerted effort to laugh as much as possible, and I'm sure my love of laughter is a big reason I've lived much longer than I was "supposed" to (more than twice as long as the statistics said I would — and I'm still going strong) after my brain tumor was diagnosed.

I'm also convinced that humor is an extremely important ingredient in a successful romantic relationship. I'm not talking about laughing at your partner, or making him or her laugh, though — I mean the ability to laugh at yourself.

Let me explain why I feel that's so important. A while ago I read about a husband whose wife made a rather snide remark about him one evening while the couple was having dinner with some friends, angrily claiming that he talked too much. Instead of blowing up at her or defending himself, the man smiled and said "You're right. I sure can dominate a conversation." As a result, a statement that could have ignited a nasty fight turned into a moment in which no damage to the relationship was done, and the husband learned something important about himself and the way others see him.

Life without hearing can be a real challenge at times, and sometimes it can be hard to laugh at anything, let alone yourself. A while ago a well-known late-deafened man remarked to me that post-lingual deafness was serious business, a sentiment I certainly share. This particular individual, however, implied it was *always* serious. I don't see it that way. Nor do I want to. Isn't there great humor in mixing up your signs and conveying a message that's very different from what you actually mean? What about doing the exact opposite of what you're asked to do because you've misunderstood the directions you were given? Wouldn't laughing about things like that be a lot better for your mental and physical health than giving yourself (or someone else) a hard time?

If you don't develop the ability to laugh at yourself or your circumstances, you're in for a very unhappy life. Your relationships, especially, will be a mess. You'll take everything far too seriously, and when your partner — who often knows you almost as well as you do — teases you or points out one of your flaws, you'll probably get angry and act defensively. You can just imagine how doing that on a regular basis can seriously damage a relationship or bring it to an end.

My "Mixed Marriage"

Although I try to laugh at myself as much as possible, there are some things I take very seriously — particularly my marriage to Marvelous Mary. She obviously cares very deeply about us too. What was it like for her when her husband went deaf? Here are her thoughts on the subject. The specifics of her reaction are undoubtedly different from that of other hearing people who are married to late-deafened individuals, although the following may strike some very familiar chords.

◆　　◆　　◆

I'm not a procrastinator. In fact, I usually plan ahead and tackle things right away. When Shawn asked me to write about our "mixed marriage," though, I couldn't seem to get started — probably because it's such an important issue for me and so hard to view through a single deaf/hearing lens when it's a complex relationship that's affected by so many factors.

On a practical level, we were very lucky. We heard of the Association of Late-Deafened Adults (ALDA) through Robin Titterington, a friend and colleague from Georgia, soon after Shawn went deaf. At our first ALDA conference in 1991, Bill Graham's future wife Karina gave me a piece of advice that I still use and share with others. This one piece of advice has probably saved my sanity as well as my relationship with Shawn. Karina told me that I was Shawn's wife — not his nurse, his interpreter, or his therapist. Remembering this, especially during the difficult times, has helped me remain focused on who I am and what my role is.

Our circumstances with Shawn's deafness are different from many couples' experience in that as a certified interpreter for the deaf, I was fluent in sign language when he lost his hearing, and had many friends in the deaf community. This, however, didn't mean that all was perfect. There were issues we still had to confront. For example, Shawn once complained that it was frustrating to him that I could sign so well and communicate so freely with other signers when he couldn't. My sign fluency also raised other issues — primarily, that I tend to sign too fast for Shawn and use sign vocabulary that he doesn't know. It's difficult for me to keep track of what signs he's familiar with and which are totally foreign to him. To deal with this, Shawn and I make sure that all our important communication is text-based. When something's significant (travel itineraries, schedules, etc.), we either send each other an e-mail or sit next to one another with a TTY or a computer and have a typed-out conversation. This helps us tremendously because through typing we're both sure that the other person understands what we're saying.

Shawn and I have also had to adjust to the more routine aspects of his hearing loss. For example, I've learned to take a key with me whenever I leave the house, even if it's just to get the mail or work in the garden. Shawn has a habit of locking the doors without looking to see if I'm on the other side. Too often I've gotten locked out of the house, and, of course, always at the most inconvenient time. One time I was barefoot on the balcony of our second story apartment in January and had to scale the outside wall to walk to a neighbor's house to call to ask Shawn to unlock the door, but Shawn, assuming I was home, waited for me to answer the telephone. So our answering machine picked up. Eventually, I did get in, but by that time I was definitely cold and more than a little cranky!

Shawn lost his hearing during the second of four brain surgeries resulting from a tumor situated on his brainstem. Essentially, he went into the second surgery hearing, and came out deaf. In and of itself, that was quite a significant issue for him to face as an individual, and for us as a couple. There were, however, other issues to deal with, such as his loss of balance, short term memory, sense of smell, and much of his eye-hand coordination, as well as the ongoing medical reality of his brain tumor. Add to this the fact that after going deaf Shawn was no longer able to remain employed, and that my income as a freelance interpreter was insufficient to support us and cover his medical costs. So we moved from Georgia to Washington, D.C. and I began working full-time at the U.S. Department of Education, first as an interpreter, then as the manager of the department's "terps," and now as a program specialist. Shawn continued his therapies and began the process of adjusting to his disabilities. He also became very active with the Association of Late-Deafened Adults and his writing, and became sort of a "house-hubby." Our lives had changed drastically.

We deal with all kinds of issues that I'm sure most other people in "mixed marriages" have experienced. First, Shawn isn't exactly a great cook, and his inability to hear or smell things doesn't help. Our neighbors laugh when our smoke alarm goes off around dinner time, because they know Shawn's cooking. If we ever have a fire between 6:00 and 7:00 p.m. nobody will help us! Second, my sisters laugh at me when I tell them I can't hear them on the telephone because Shawn's putting away the pots and pans and has forgotten that they make noise when they're banged together. Third, Shawn and I have had to agree that he can- not vacuum after I go to bed! He forgets that certain appliances make noise and can wake me up. Finally, the cats and bunny have had to get used to his "noisy" movements. The list goes on, but I'm sure you get the picture.

This works both ways, though: Shawn has to deal with my hearing-ness too. He has to see me communicate easily with others, use the telephone in the usual way, and enjoy the sounds of music and nature. I also can't sign to him if I have my hands full of grocery bags or other items. I can't always talk while driving either, especially when I have to negotiate a busy intersection. Traffic and sledge hammers also make noise and interfere with my ability to hear him when he talks, even if he can't hear them. I love the sounds of things, such as Christmas carols, waterfalls, ocean waves, and birds chirping, and sometimes need to enjoy the auditory environment we live in. I wish he could too.

Through all of this, though, our love and determination ("stubbornness" may be a more accurate term!) have gotten us through these moments and through the tough times in our relationship. We try to maintain a sense of humor about what happens, and remember that our unique perspectives are both valid. It's not always easy, but we're never bored!

◆   ◆   ◆

So there you have it — some of the joys and challenges my wife and I share. I imagine they're not all that different from the ones that many other people in "mixed marriages" deal with.

Think About All the Things Your Significant Other Does

As I said in the section about forgetting traditional gender roles, I'm kind of a house-hubby now. My wife goes to work, and I stay home. When I'm not writing or exercising, I take care of most of the day-to-day chores, such as shopping, cooking, and cleaning. Although doing certain things can be tricky for me because of my terrible balance and coordination, I still manage to do quite a bit (hey, Mary got it at least half right when she said we were a very stubborn couple, because her husband sure is!).

A while ago, though, I realized that how much I do doesn't compare to everything Mary does. She works full-time, so we can put food on the table and pay the bills, went to school part-time for five years to get her Masters degree, and has to keep up with her domestic obligations and friendships. On top of it all, she's tremendously loving and supportive of me. At times I find myself stopping and simply giving thanks for all the things she does, both for me and for us as a couple. I often wonder how I ever got so lucky.

I also make an effort to regularly express my gratitude to Mary for everything she does. Late-deafened people with hearing spouses or significant others might want do the same. It's not always readily apparent, but hearing spouses of late-deafened people are often some of the busiest people around. In my own case, my wife is often my interpreter, especially in my relationships with friends and relatives, works full time, and attends many of the conferences and social events I go to.

I suspect that sort of thing is true for a lot of late-deafened people. Yet many of us, especially if we've been married or in a monogamous relationship for a long time, tend to forget all the things our significant other does for us. Why not change that? Stop thinking about all the things you do and start focusing on the things your partner does for you and both of you. Then show your gratitude for that — whether though little gifts, kind words, or both. You'll be amazed at how much that changes your attitude towards your loved one and the relationship you share.

Love On-line

One of the greatest benefits of the modern age is that computers have made it easier to do so many things. We can download and send documents that look great even if our typing is less than wonderful, buy virtually anything we want, and find almost any kind of information we need by visiting the right site and simply clicking our mouse.

The biggest question for many late-deafened computer users, though, may be this: "can we find love on-line?" The answer is a resounding "yes."

The greatest advantage of on-line romance for late-deafened people is quite obvious: when we're looking for love electronically our inability to hear doesn't matter. If we can read, we can understand exactly what the other person is saying. We also don't have to worry about being misunderstood by the other party (a concern for late-deafened people who don't sign well or those who have — like me — a voice that's hard to understand), because our thoughts and feelings are very clearly expressed in type.

There are also benefits to on-line romance that go beyond the issue of understanding what's said. When we meet someone in person, we usually evaluate (whether consciously or subconsciously) his or her looks right away. Only later do we form an opinion of what that person is really like. But when we meet people on-line, it's just the opposite. We have no idea what the person we're talking with looks like, and it's his or her mind we encounter first. We may eventually meet that person in the flesh, and evaluate his or her looks, but before we do that we get to know how he or she feels and thinks. As a result, on-line relationships can be considerably stronger than traditional ones because the emphasis is on the mind and the spirit rather than physical appearance.

How serious can an on-line relationship become? That depends on many factors, but they can be condensed into a couple important considerations:

- Do you "play it safe" in on-line relationships, or do you use (and expect) honesty and frankness? The latter will lead to a much more meaningful relationship than the former.

- Do you really get to know the other person? Does he or she get to know you well? Or do both of you hide who you really are? The latter wll result in a cautious and lukewarm relationship, while the former can produce something much more intense and satisfying.

It's also a good idea to learn as much as possible about the person you interact with before meeting him or her in person. For many people that means doing some research or hiring a private detective. The Internet, unfortunately, seems to have become a haven for false advertising and dishonesty, and you don't want to fall victim to either when interacting with a possible mate.

Critics of on-line relationships often condemn them as superficial or inconsequential because they lack the physical element that's prevalent in so many traditional romances. Judging from the relationships I've seen between late-deafened people who met on-line and then in person, though, there's nothing shallow about them.

A RESOURCE RESOURCE

Although going deaf is no fun (how's that for an understatement?), there are lots of resources available to help make the transition to a silent world easier. The following isn't meant to be an exhaustive listing of what's available for late-deafened people, it can at least point you in the right direction. Some of the resources listed below have appeared in previous chapters or are included in more than one section of this listing, so don't be too concerned if you get a sense of déjà vú when you read them.

T=TTY, V=Voice, F=Facsimile, E=E-mail, I=Internet

<u>Organizations</u>

At the top of my list of valuable resources for late-deafened people is the Association of Late-Deafened Adults (ALDA), which offers information about acquired deafness and support for individuals who are late-deafened. Membership in ALDA (currently $20/year) includes a subscription to *ALDA News*, the organization's quarterly newsletter. The group also holds a yearly conference in various cities, and has local chapters and groups throughout the United States and the world. You can learn more about ALDA at the following addresses and numbers.

> Association of Late-Deafened Adults
> 131 Lake Street #204
> Oak Park, IL 60301
> (708) 358-0135 (T)
> (877) 907-1738 (V, F)
> info@alda.org (E)
> www.alda.org (I)

Although its focus in recent years has been on Deaf people rather than those who went deaf post-lingually, Hearing Loss Link — which was started by ALDA co-founder Bill Graham and his wife Karina — provides assistance for deaf and deafened individuals throughout the United States.

> Hearing Loss Link
> 2001 N. Clybourn Avenue, 2nd Floor
> Chicago, IL 60614
> (773) 248-9174 (T)
> (773) 248-9121(V)
> (773) 248-9176 (F)
> http://www.hearinglosslink.org/(I)

Many people who lose most but not all of their hearing consider themselves hard of hearing rather than deaf, and want to focus on maximizing the hearing they still have. If you fit that description, you might want to check out:

> Self Help for Hard of Hearing People, Inc. (SHHH)
> 7910 Woodmont Ave., Suite 1200
> Bethesda, MD 20814
> (301) 657-2249 (T)
> (301) 657-2248 (V)
> (301) 913-9413 (F)
> national@shhh.org (E)
> http://www.shhh.org (I)

Are you an African-American with less-than-perfect hearing? If so, you might want to learn more about this organization:

> National Black Deaf Advocates
> Times Square
> P.O. Box 2021
> New York, New York 10108
> Syounger 64@hotmail.com (E)
> http://www.ndba.org/index.html (I)

It may not qualify as an organization since it's just one small part of Gallaudet University, but the National Information Center on Deafness (NICD) might be just what you're looking for. It's a great source of information and referrals that can help you a lot (I'm a *little* biased because I used to volunteer at the NICD, and love the place!). You can find out more about the university and the NICD by contacting:

Gallaudet University
800 Florida Ave NE
Washington, DC 20002-3695
(202) 651-5052 (T)
(202) 651-5051 (V)
(202) 651-5054 (F)
http://www.gallaudet.edu/(I)

Simple conversation, so common in the hearing world, can be hard to come by when you're late-deafened. But a pair of men who lost their hearing as adults, both former members of the ALDA board of directors, have filled the void by creating on-line lists called "The SayWhatClub," the brainstorm of Bob Elkins, and "LDA Chat" an electronic gem founded by former ALDA president Ken Arcia. On both services subscribers talk about everything from deafness to recipes, and offer jokes, riddles, and just about anything else you can imagine. If you'd like to find out more about either of them, head to the following WWW addresses.

The SayWhatClub
http://www.saywhatclub.com/(I)

LDA Chat
http://groups.yahoo.com/group/LDAchat/(I)

Tinnitus

A late-deafened man once told me that dealing with his tinnitus, which is often referred to as "head noise" or "ringing in the ears," and isn't uncommon among late-deafened people, was "like living in the rear of a jet." Really funny, but very true, as many people with tinnitus can tell you. If you'd like to learn more about the subject, you can contact the American Tinnitus Association at:

ATA National Headquarters
PO Box 5
Portland, OR 97207-0005
(800) 634-8978 (V) [Toll Free within the U.S.]
(503) 248-9985 (V)
(503) 248-0024 (F)

tinnitus@ata.org (E)
http://www.ata.org/about_ata/contact.html (I)

Neurofibromatosis

Want to learn more about neurofibromatotis, a disease that's often a cause of acquired deafness? Start by contacting one of the following organizations:

Neurofibromatotis, Inc
8855 Annapolis Road, Suite 110
Lanham, MD 20706-2924
(800) 942-6825 (V)
(301) 918-4600 (V)
(301) 918-0009 (F)

The National Neurofibromatosis Foundation, Inc.
95 Pine Street, 16th Floor
New York, NY 10005
(212) 344-6633 (V)
(800) 323-7938 (Toll-Free V)
NNFF@nf.org (E)
(212) 747-0004 (F)
http://www.nf.org/contact_us/(I)

You can also chat online about the illness with members of the "NF-2 Crew." To find out more about the Crew — started by late-deafened people with the disease — point your browser at htttp://www.webcrossings.com/nf2crew/(I)

Other Medical Resources

For questions about hearing or speech, a great starting point is the American Speech-Language-Hearing Association, which can be reached at the following number and addresses.

American Speech-Language-Hearing Association
10801 Rockville Pike
Rockville, MD 20852
(800) 638-8255(T, V)
action.center@asha.org (E)
http://www.asha.org/about/contacts.cfm (I)

Want to learn more about head and neck surgery, which is often a major concern for late-deafened people who lose their hearing because of medical problems? Contact the American Academy of Otolaryngology.

American Academy of Otolaryngology
Head and Neck Surgery
1 Prince Street
Alexandria, VA 22314
(703) 836-4444 (V)
http://www.si.umich.edu/HCHS (I)

Legal Concerns

If you're wondering about your rights as a deaf person and what the Americans with Disabilities Act can do for you, you can get answers at:

U.S. Department of Justice
950 Pennsylvania Avenue, NW
Civil Rights Division

National Council on Disability
1331 F St. NW, Ste. 850
Washington, D.C.
800/877-8339 (T)
202/272-2004 (V)

Federal Communications Commission
445 12th Street, SW
Washington, D.C. 20554
(888) 835-5322 (T, toll-free)
(888) 225-5322 (V, toll-free)
(202) 418-2555 (T)
(202) 418-2830 (F on demand)
http://www.fcc.gov/contacts.html (I)
fccinfo@fcc.gov (E)

Captioning

As I pointed out in the chapter about daily life for late-deafened people, one of the greatest boons for late-deafened people in the past few years is the growth of both closed- and open-captioning, which allow people to read rather than hear the spoken dialogue of a television program, commercial, movie, or play. There are many different firms that provide captioning services. Two of the best are The National Captioning Institute and Caption First. You can find out more about captioning from both of them.

National Captioning Institute
333 Seventh Avenue, 10th Floor
New York, NY 10001
(212) 557-7011 (T/V)
(212) 557-6975 F)
mail@ncicap.org (E)

Caption First
3238 Rose Street
Franklin Park, IL 60131
(847) 451-7508 (T)
(847) 451-7397 or (800) 825-5235(V)
(847) 451-7504 (F)
info@captionfirst.com (E)
http://www.captionfirst.com/overview.htm (I)

Education

If you're interested in either complete degree programs or individual courses, you might want to consider one of the following:

Gallaudet University
800 Florida Avenue NE
Washington, DC 20002
(202) 651-5000 (T/V)
http://www.gallaudet.edu/(I)

Rochester Institute of Technology
National Technical Institute for the Deaf
Lyndon Baines Johnson Building
52 Lomb Memorial Drive
Rochester, NY 14623-5604
585) 475-6400 (T, V)
(585) 475-5623 (F)

NTIDMC@rit.edu (E)
www.rit.edu/NTID (I)

As I pointed out in the chapter about daily life for late-deafened people, other options for deafened individuals in search of education are on-line and correspondence courses, since neither require a sense of hearing. You can also see if there's a correspondence course available in your area of interest or an on-line course that focuses on a subject you want to know more about.

Psychology

If you'd like to learn more about the psychology of late-deafness, you might want to get in touch with the California School of Professional Psychology (CSPP), which is now a part of Alliant International University. To learn more about the various CSPP programs that are available, contact:

Alliant International University
Continuing Education Division
2728 Hyde Street, Suite 100
San Francisco, CA 94109-1252
(800) 467-1273 (V)
admissions@alliant.edu (E)
http://www.alliant.edu/ce/(I)

Hearing Aids and Cochlear Implants

As I pointed out in the chapters about hearing aids and cochlear implants, many late-deafened individuals rely on them to hear better. If you'd like to learn more about either or both, you certainly won't lack for organizations that provide information on the subjects. Two of the best are:

Alexander Graham Bell Association for the Deaf
3417 Volta Place, NW
Washington, DC 20007-2778
(202) 337-5220 (V/T)
(800) 432-7543 (Toll Free)
(202) 337-8314 (F)
AGBELL2@aol.com (E)
www.agbell.org (I)

American Academy of Audiology
8300 Greensboro Drive, Suite 750
Mclean, VA 22102-3611
(703) 610-9022 (V/T)
(800) AAA-2336 (Toll Free)
(703) 610-9005 (F)
www.audiology.org (I)

If you're specifically interested in cochlear implants, you can check with your doctor or do an online search using words like "cochlear implants," which will provide you with the names and website addresses of companies that manufacture cochlear implants. A late-deafened woman who uses a cochlear implant also suggested a website called CIHear on Yahoo Groups, in which members share information about implants without the pressure or self-congratulation usually found on websites or e-mail list run by producers of C.I.s. The website's address is

http://groups.yahoo.com/group/CIHear/

You might also want to check out another on-line club that focuses on cochlear implants:

Cochlear Implant Club International
5335 Wisconsin Ave. NW, Suite 440
Washington, D.C. 20015-2003
(202) 895-2781 (T/V)
(202) 895-2782 (F)
http://www.skypoint.com/~samtd/xyzcici/

There are also a number of books about implants. As I said at the start of the chapter about cochear implants, I'm particularly fond of Bev Biderman's book Wired for Sound: A Journey Into Hearing. Late-deafened individuals who are considering getting a cochlear implant can also look at Hear Again: Back to Life with a Cochlear Implant by Arlene Rom-off, who began losing her hearing as a college student and was eventually left profoundly deaf. She then got a C.I., and in the book talks about the very positive results she got from it.

Hearing Dogs

The chapter on assistive devices talks about getting a canine pal that will run back and forth, jump up and down, or otherwise notify its owner when it hears the phone ring, a smoke alarm go off, and much more. There are many non-profit organizations that provide hearing dogs at little or no charge. If you'd like more information on the subject, contact:

> Dogs for the Deaf
> 10175 Wheeler Road
> Central Point, OR 97502
> (541) 876-9220 (T, V)
> (541) 876-6696 (F)
> info@dogsforthedeaf.org (E)
> http://www.dogsfor the deaf.org/top.htm (I)

The Americans with Disabilities Act

The chapter about the Americans with Disabilities Act (ADA) talked about the many benefits the act provides. If you'd like to learn more about specific aspects of the ADA, the following offices, departments, and commissions can help.

> Architectural and Transportation Barriers
> Compliance Board
> 1331 F Street, NW Suite 1000
> Washington, D.C. 22036-3894
> (800) 872-2253 (T/V)
> (202) 272-5449 (T)

> Department of Justice
> Office of the Americans with Disabilities Act
> Civil Rights Division
> P.O. Box 66118
> Washington, D.C. 20530

> Department of Transportation
> 400 Seventh Street, SW
> Washington, D.C. 20590

(202) 755-7687 (T)
202) 366-9305 (V)

Federal Communications Commission
1919 M Street, NW
Washing999 (T)
(202) 632-7260 (V)

Employment

If you're specifically interested in the employment aspects of the ADA, you'll want to contact the U.S. Equal Employment Opportunity Commission (EEOC) at:

U.S. Equal Employment Opportunity Commission
1801 L Street, N.W.
Washington, D.C. 20507
(202) 663-4494 (T)
(202) 663-4900 (V)

There are also regional EEOC offices in many large cities. Check your phone book to see if there's one near you.

Another excellent resource for late-deafened people who want to work is the President's Committee on the Employment of People with Disabilities. Contact the commission at:

President's Committee on the Employment
of People with Disabilities
1331 F Street, NW
Washington, DC 20004-1107
(202) 376-6205 (T)
(202) 376-6200 (V)
(202) 376-6219 (F)

Last, but certainly not least, is the Job Accommodation Network (JAN), run by the U.S Department of Labor, which offers information about the Americans with Disabilities Act and the employment of disabled people. To learn more about the JAN, contact the Department at:

U.S. Department of Labor
200 Constitution Ave., NW

Washington, DC 20210
1-866-889-5627 (T)
1-866-4-USA-DOL (V)

You can also get in touch with the JAN directly by calling:

1-800-526-7234 (T, V)

Travel

If you'd like to learn more about traveling after a hearing loss, read Joan Cassidy's excellent travel tips in the Daily Life chapter. For travel to Europe, you might want to contact either:

Tripscop
63 Esmond Road
London, W4 1JE
United Kingdom
44-81-994-9294 (V)

or

Comité national français de liaison pour la réadaptation des handicappés

38, Boulevard Raspaic,
75007, Paris, France
45-48-90-13 (V)

Written Material

If you're reading this book, you're obviously interested in written material about late-deafness. Following are some works on the subject.

Books

Himber, Charlotte. How to Survive Hearing Loss

Written by a woman who lost much of her hearing later in life, this book focuses primarily on reduced hearing due to aging. Himber refers to several devices — hearing aids, TTYs, assistive listening devices, and so on — that can be helpful to anyone determined to live as fully as possible after a hearing loss.

Dugan, Marcia B., <u>Living with Hearing Loss</u>

This helpful book discusses many issues persons with a hearing loss and their families should know about, and provides information on cochlear implants and tinnitus. It also offers information about hearing-related Internet sites and a listing of resources for making it easier to deal with hearing loss. Its focus, however, is largely on mild or moderate hearing loss, so the book is more appropriate for individuals who consider themselves hard of hearing rather than deaf.

Jones, Leslie, Jim Kyle, and Peter Woods, eds. <u>Words Apart</u>

<u>Words Apart</u> provides an exhaustive look at the social and psychological aspects of late-deafness. Edited by three Britons, <u>Words Apart</u> is a detailed investigation of hearing loss and ways to overcome many of its challenges.

Kaplan, Harriet, Scott Bally, and Carol Garretson. <u>Speechreading: A Way to Improve Understanding</u>

A detailed look at the role of speechreading in assisting the comprehension of spoken words, <u>Speechreading: A Way to Improve Understanding</u> discusses the history of speechreading, its general principles, and the advantages and limitations of speechreading in everyday life. The book also provides exercises on various speechreading techniques that allow the reader to practice on his or her own and with others.

Orlans, Harold (editor). <u>Adjustment to Adult Hearing Loss</u>

This 12-chapter volume contains essays and articles about various social and psychological aspects of late-deafness. Each chapter is written by a different individual, and looks at various issues of acquired deafness, ranging from Orlans' own "Reflections on Adult Hearing Loss" to Pauline Ashley's "Deafness in the Family," the story of the acquired deafness of her husband, Jack Ashley, who was a member of the British parliament when he lost his hearing.

<u>Adjustment to Adult Hearing Loss</u> includes the following chapters:

Ashley, Jack A. "A Personal Account."

This chapter presents Ashley's personal view of his battle with adult-onset deafness and his decision to remain in the British parliament after losing his hearing. While not as extensive as his book <u>Journey Into Silence</u>, Ashley's "A Personal Account" provides a first-hand view of the obstacles and challenges the author faced after going deaf.

Ashley, Pauline K. "Deafness in the Family."

Written by the wife of Jack Ashley, this chapter describes how her husband's late-deafness influenced his life both in Parliament and at home. The author talks about how her husband dealt with several areas of concern, including telephone usage after going deaf and learning speechreading.

Meadow-Orlans, Kathryn. "Social and Psychological Effects of Hearing Loss in Adult hood: A Literature Review."

Meadow-Orlans looks at the particular challenges faced by individuals who are late-deafened, pointing out that they have often been lumped with the culturally Deaf. She also notes the lack of written material on acquired deafness, writes about the psychological influences of hearing loss (paranoia, depression, and nervousness, among other things), and addresses the social changes that often accompany it. Meadow-Orlans also devotes a section of this piece to hearing loss among the elderly. The chapter combines a review of the research literature available on late-deafness with insights drawn from the author's personal experiences.

Orlans, Harold. "Reflections on Adult Hearing Loss."

In summing up his book on hearing loss, Orlans offers some wise observations about the lack of organizations representing the needs of the late-deafened, and the small amount of psychological study that's been done on adult-onset deafness. Orlans also looks at the regrettable lack of interaction between Deaf, deaf, hard of hearing, late-deafened, and hearing individuals, and offers a definition of the term "accepting deafness."

Oyer, Herbert J. and E. Jane Oyer. "Adult Hearing Loss and the Family."

This piece looks at the family of an adult who loses his or her hearing, and the rehabilitation of deafened individuals. The authors talk about theoretical approaches in family research — the developmental and the crisis-oriented models in particular — and how the family copes with a member's acquired deafness. They also consider the impact of acquired deafness on one's friends, and present a theoretical model of hearing impairment and family relationships.

Rezen, Susan and Carl Hausman. "Coping with Hearing Loss: A Guide for Adults and Their Families."

"Coping with Hearing Loss" offers a comprehensive view of post-lingual hearing loss, and how it can affect both individuals with the loss and their families, friends, and acquaintances. The book looks at the loss of hearing among both elderly and younger people, and suggests practical and psychological strategies for living a full and satisfying life after a hearing loss.

Canadian Hard-of-Hearing Association Life After Deafness: A Resource Book for Late-Deafened Adults

This book contains several addresses and pieces of information that are relevant to Canadians, but is also full of tips and facts that apply to all late-deafened people, regardless of where they live.

Thomsett, Kay, and Eva Nickerson. Missing Words: The Family Handbook on Adult Hearing Loss

The combined effort of a late-deafened former schoolteacher, Eva Nickerson, and her daughter Kay Thomsett, a writer/editor in the U.S. Department of Veterans' Affairs, Missing Words suggests several practical steps a person can take after experiencing a hearing loss. Much of the book's advice centers on speechreading and how best to live in the hearing world as a post-lingually deaf person. The book also includes information about cochlear implant and hearing aid use, which is provided by Nickerson's otolaryngologist, Donald H. Holden, M.D.

Woodcock, Kathryn and Miguel Aguayo. Deafened People: Adjustment and Support

Written by two late-deafened adults, Deafened People is a very valuable resource for those who are interested in the psychological aspect of adult-onset hearing loss. Despite its rather formal tone and very high retail price ($21.95 for the paperback version and $60.00 for the hardback one), the book provides lots of helpful information about the emotional aspect of late-deafness.

Articles

There are a number of articles that address subjects of interest to late-deafened people. While I couldn't possibly list all of them here (that could be a book in and of itself!) I encourage you to look at the following periodicals to find pieces of interest to you. "ALDA News," "American Annals of the Deaf," "British Journal of Audiology," "Hearing Health," "Hearing Loss" (formerly known as "SHHH Journal"), "NAD Mag" and the previously-mentioned on-line periodical "HOH-LD-News."

GLOSSARY

Adventitiously deaf: Persons with little or no hearing because of unknown causes, illness, or accident.

ALD: Assistive Listening Device.

ALDA: Association of Late-Deafened Adults. Founded in 1987, ALDA lobbies for the needs of late-deafened people and provides them with social and educational opportunities.

American Sign Language (ASL): A visual-gestural language used by many Deaf people, ASL has its own vocabulary and sentence structure, and is a language unto itself rather than a simple translation of spoken English into sign language.

Assistive devices: Assistive devices (TTY's, visual and vibro tactile alarm clocks, baby cry alarms, and so on) take advantage of senses besides hearing to help deaf or hard of hearing people continue to live their daily lives without relying on the use of their hearing.

Assistive listening devices: Often called ALDs, Assistive Listening Devices — such as hearing aids, amplifiers, and FM loops — magnify the sounds they receive so that people with residual hearing can maximize their ability to understand what's been said or hear sounds around them.

Audiogram: An audiogram is a graph showing the degree of loudness at which a person hears a sound of a particular frequency ("frequency" is defined below).

Audiologically deaf: This term is used to describe a physical state. Some people who lose their hearing post-lingually erroneously describe themselves as "Deaf" with a capital "D," which refers to a specific cultural identity rather than a medical condition.

Audiologist: A healthcare specialist who measures an individual's hearing ability and provides information about different assistive listening devices.

Auditory Brainstem Implant (ABI): An alternative to cochlear implants, an ABI bypasses the cochlea altogether. Its electrode is connected directly to the base of the brain. A very limited number of hospitals and medical centers are authorized to implant ABI's. Many individuals receiving an ABI are NF-2 patients having surgery for the removal of a second tumor.

Auditory nerve: The auditory nerve is a cranial nerve that carries information from the inner ear to the brain.

Aural rehabilitation: Training in procedures that will improve communication skills.

CART: This is an abbreviation for the term "Computer Assisted RealTime" or "Computer Assisted Realtime Transcription" a form of communication that allows spoken words to appeal on a screen so deaf people can read them. CART is very popular among late-deafened people.

CICI: Cochlear Implant Club International (CICI) is a group that provides support and information to people with cochlear implants and those who want to know more about them. It can be reached at (202) 895-2781 (T/V), (202) 895-2782 (F), http://www.skypoint.com/~samtd/xyzcici/(I).

Closed captions: The on-screen display of dialogue (and occasionally other sounds) of a captioned television show, movie, or commercial. Closed captions are seen through an internal decoder chip in a television or an external decoder mechanism. Televisions with a diagonal screen measure of 13 inches or larger sold in the United States after July 1, 1993 were required to contain a decoder chip that allowed the viewing of closed captions with a simple adjustment.

Cochlea: Shaped like a snail shell, the cochlea is the hearing part of the inner ear.

Cochlear Implant (CI): A surgically-implanted device which stimulates the auditory fibers of the inner ear and allows deaf individuals to process certain auditory information.

Communication Assistant (CA): A Telephone Relay Service (see below) employee who serves as the "ears" for TTY-using individuals when speaking by telephone with a hearing individual or business that does not have a TTY.

Conductive hearing loss: A hearing loss caused by an abnormality in the middle or outer ear.

Cued Speech: Cued speech augments the words of a speaker by providing a series of handshape cues to enable speechreaders to distinguish among sounds that look similar on the lips.

Culturally Deaf: Those who were born deaf or lost their hearing at a young age, and use sign language as their principle means of communication. Culturally Deaf children often attend a special school for deaf students, although the number who are "mainstreamed" (i.e. attend public or private schools where teachers and students are hearing) has grown markedly in recent years.

Deaf and deaf: A capital "D" in the word "deaf" refers to a cultural state, while a lower-case "d" indicates a physical condition in which a person has little or no ability to hear, but isn't culturally Deaf.

Decibel (dB): Decibels measure the loudness of a sound. People with normal hearing can hear sounds at 25 decibels or fewer. Those with a hearing loss are classified by the volume required for them to hear a sound: a person with a mild loss can hear a sound of 26–40 dB, those with a moderate loss can hear sounds from 41–55 dB, people who hear sounds from 71–90 dB are considered severally impaired, and those who are profoundly deaf need sounds to be more than 90 dB in order to hear them. The "B" in dB is capitalized in honor of Alexander Graham Bell, a strong advocate for deaf and hard of hearing people and an outspoken supporter of the oral approach to communication for them.

Ear, nose, and throat doctor (ENT): Also called an otolaryngologist or otologist (and sometimes even an otorhinolaryngologist!), an ENT is a physician who specializes in ear, nose, and throat problems.

Fingerspelling: In this mode of communication, often used by signers when there is no sign language equivalent for a given word or the sign is unknown, the word is spelled out using an individual handshape for each letter in it.

FM system: An FM system transmits a signal by way of radio waves sent from the sound source to an individual listener wearing a receiver. FM systems are particularly useful in auditoriums, because their signals have a range of more than 100 yards and can pass through physical obstructions.

Frequency: Frequency is measured in terms of the number of complete cycles a sound makes in a unit of time. The higher the pitch of a sound, the greater its frequency.

Hair cells: Hair cells are receptors in the cochlea that translate sound vibrations into messages which are then sent to the brain via the auditory nerve.

Hard of hearing (HOH): People who are hard of hearing are generally members of mainstream society, but don't hear perfectly and usually supplement their hearing with hearing aids and other assistive listening devices.

Hearing aids: Worn in the ear, behind it, and, less frequently now, on the body, hearing aids amplify all sounds they receive. Most hearing aids allow the user to determine to what extent sounds of various frequencies are amplified.

Hertz (Hz): A scientific unit used for the measurement of frequency.

Induction loop system: See audio loop system

Infrared system: Often used in theaters, this is a system in which a transmitter broadcasts a signal using invisible infrared light waves.

Lipreading: See speechreading

Manual deaf: Also called manualists, the manual deaf are individuals who use some form of sign language as their principal means of communication.

Manually Coded English (MCE): Embracing sign systems that present words in English word order, and often including articles such as "the" and "a," MCE usually includes Pidgin Signed English, Signed Exact English I and II, Conceptually Accurate Signed English, and Seeing Exact English.

Meniere's Disease: This illness usually causes loud noises in the ears, vertigo or dizziness, and a sense of fullness in the head. Marked by an over accumulation of fluid in the inner ear, Meniere's Disease sometimes leads to hearing loss.

Meningitis: A disease which sometimes causes a person to lose his or her hearing, meningitis is an illness of the spinal cord or brain.

Neurofibromatosis (NF): A genetic neurological disorder that can cause deafness, neurofibromatosis is divided into two categories: NF-1 (formerly called Recklinghausen's Disease), and NF-2. The former is characterized by tumors that appear on the outside of the body, while the latter causes internal tumors which sometimes develop on the brain and can lead to hearing and balance problems.

Open captions: Similar to subtitles, open captions appear at the top or bottom of a television or movie screen and can be read without a decoder.

Oral deaf: This term refers to deaf persons who use speech and speech-reading to communicate instead of sign language. Oral deaf individuals are sometimes called "Oralists."

Otitis Media: Often caused by an infection, otitis media is an inflammation of the middle ear that can lead to deafness.

Otology: The study of the anatomy and diseases of the ear.

Ototoxic: Used to refer to certain drugs, such as some antibiotics, "oto-toxic" literally means "poisonous to the ear."

Presbycusis: A sensorineural hearing loss that accompanies aging.

Residual Hearing: Hearing retained by deaf, Deaf, and hard of hearing people.

Sensorineural Hearing Loss: A hearing loss resulting from damage to, or alteration of, the sensory mechanisms of the cochlea or the neural structures of the inner ear and brain.

Sign Language: This name is used to denote any system of communication that uses hand configurations and gestures as the principal means of expression.

Speechreading: Sometimes called "lipreading," speechreading is the ability to understand spoken words by observing the speaker's lips, gestures, expressions, and body language.

TDD: See TTY

Telephone Relay Service (TRS): With many options of interest to late-deafened people, a TRS acts as the "ears" for deaf and hard of hearing people and facilitates telephone contact between them and people who are hearing. A TRS has traditionally been used with a telephone, although there are now a growing number of on-line relay services that call for the use of a computer rather than a phone.

Tinnitus: Sometimes called "head noise" or "ringing in the ears," tinnitus is any sound heard only by a single individual and not resulting from an external stimulus. Many late-deafened people have to deal with tinnitus, which can take the form of ringing in the ears, chirping, clicking, whistling, roaring, or hissing.

T-switch: Many hearing aids have a T-switch (the "T" stands for "Telecoil" or "Telephone"), which can pick up magnetic fields generated by electronic devices, audio loop systems, and hearing-aid-compatible telephones.

TTY (sometimes called a TDD or TT): TTY stands for "Teletypewriter," TDD means "Telecommunications Device for the Deaf," and TT is the abbreviation for "Text Telephone." All three terms signify the same thing — a machine with a keyboard and a small screen which allows deaf and hard of hearing people to use the telephone by reading what the other party or a TRS communication assistant (see above) types.

Vocational Rehabilitation: The evaluation and training or retraining of individuals for work opportunities.

978-0-595-30661-9
0-595-30661-6

Printed in the United States
33263LVS00006B/16